ESSENTIAL AUDIOLOGY FOR PHYSICIANS

A Singular Audiology Text

Jeffrey L. Danhauer, Ph.D.

Audiology Editor

ESSENTIAL AUDIOLOGY FOR PHYSICIANS

Kathleen Campbell, PhD

Professor and Director of Audiology
Southern Illinois University
School of Medicine
Springfield, Illinois

Singular Publishing Group, Inc.
San Diego • London

Singular Publishing Group, Inc.
401 West A Street, Suite 325
San Diego, California 92101-7904

Singular Publishing Ltd.
19 Compton Terrace
London N1 2UN, UK

e-mail: singpub@mail.cerfnet.com
Website: http://www.singpub.com

Typeset in 10/12 Palatino by Artmania!
Printed in the United States of America by Bang Printing
Second Printing 11/98

Library of Congress Cataloging-in-Publication Data
Campbell, Kathleen. 1952-
     Essential audiology for physicians / Kathleen Campbell
        p.   cm.
     Includes bibliographical references and index.
     ISBN 1-56595-691-4
     1. Audiology.   I. Title
     [DNLM: 1. Audiology.   WV 270 C188e 1997]
RF290.C35 1997
617.8--dc21
DNLM/DLC
for Library of Congress   97-34544
                                                       CIP

CONTENTS

PREFACE

Over the years, one of my favorite activities has been teaching physicians of various specialties, particularly residents, about audiology. One of the frustrations, however, is that they have frequently asked for a concise book outlining the core information they needed, but none was available. Specifically, they wanted an inexpensive paperback book that they could read quickly, yet that would provide them with the essential information, including the acronyms and abbreviations, they needed to be familiar with for clinical work. There are many excellent texts emphasizing various aspects of audiology but most are too detailed for introductory reading by busy physicians.

With changes in health care, an increasing number of physicians need to be familiar with audiologic tests, terminology, result interpretation, and options for patient management. Therefore, this book is written not only for otolaryngologists but also for physicians in primary care, neurology, pediatrics, neonatology, and physicians seeing patients on ototoxic medications such as infectious disease specialists and oncologists. Because some managed care companies now require referral by CPT code, a special CPT code index is provided. Therefore managed care companies may find this text useful in their reviews and decisions on utilization of audiologic services.

It should be noted that this book is not intended to cover all the areas or parameters of audiologic practice. Instead it covers only the information that physicians generally need to know to interact effectively with audiologists. The references and recommended readings section are limited to those directly applicable to the information that may be "essential" for physicians. Whenever possible, general overview materials are listed rather than an extensive listing of individual studies because these are usually the materials sought by physicians first learning about audiology.

This book evolved from my lecture series with the otolaryngology residents. Each chapter was distributed to them in advance of each lecture. They then reviewed each chapter, answered the self-assessment questions, reviewed the answers, and then provided me with feedback and suggestions for each chapter. Their contributions and enthusiasm significantly strengthened, and streamlined, this book. Therefore, I would like to thank Marty Janning MD, JudyAnn Krenning MD, Andrea Kittrell MD, Kurt Korver MD, John Touliatos

MD, and Jim Kalkanis MD for their review and input. Hopefully, their good scores on the inservice exam's audiology section have served as some partial repayment for their efforts. The continued commitment of Horst Konrad MD, Chairman of Otolaryngology, and Roland Folse MD, Chairman of Surgery, to physician education must also be acknowledged.

In addition to the residents' review, I asked colleagues of mine to review selected chapters. Special appreciation is extended to Nancy Tye-Murray, PhD, Lucille Beck, PhD, and Alice E. Holmes, PhD. I would also like to thank Jeffrey Danhauer, PhD, my editor at Singular Publishing, for his prompt and excellent review of each chapter. From our first conversation regarding this book, we were in complete agreement on its purpose and design. It has been truly a pleasure to work with him. I would also like to thank Larry Mazzeo, MS, and Steve Test, CNE, MCSE, for their assistance with computer graphics.

Finally, I would like to thank my husband Craig, the most enthusiastic and supportive of husbands.

The Basic Audiologic Assessment

OVERVIEW: This chapter describes the basic audiologic assessement and interpretation including the audiogram, common speech tests, and types and degrees of hearing loss. Special considerations including masking, masking dilemmas, shadow curves, and the occlusion effect are discussed. A list of abbreviations used in test reports is included.

THE AUDIOGRAM

The audiogram is a graph with frequency plotted on the X axis and intensity on the Y axis. Unlike most graphs, the Y axis is plotted from the lowest intensity at the top of the graph and the highest intensity at the bottom and frequency is listed across the top, rather than the bottom of the graph.

Stimulus frequency is plotted in **Hertz (Hz)** which is cycles per second. The frequencies included in the conventional audiogram do not cover the entire range of human hearing (usually considered as 20 to 20,000 Hz), but rather the range of hearing considered to be essential for understanding speech (250 to 8000 Hz). Other frequencies may contribute to speech understanding (and even within this range, some frequencies are more important than others), but the 250 to 8000 Hz range is commonly used.

Intensity is plotted in **decibels (dB) hearing level (HL)** rather than **sound pressure level (SPL)**. HL is based on a reference of normal human hearing threshold for each frequency, while SPL is based on an absolute pressure measurement. Therefore, the two are not equivalent. Because human hearing is not linear, at some frequencies we need greater sound intensity (in SPL) to reach threshold than at other frequencies. The HL scale normalizes these values so that 0 dB HL at 250 Hz and 0 dB HL at 1000 Hz both represent the threshold of normal human hearing at each frequency. However, greater signal intensity, as measured in SPL, will be required to reach the 0 dB HL threshold level at 250 Hz than at 1000 Hz.

An audiogram represents the behavioral responses of the patient. Normal adults and older children, can respond by raising a hand or pushing a button whenever a sound is detected. Threshold is considered as the point where the patient can just detect the signal 50% of the time.

Air-conduction responses are tested under earphone as the signal passes from the outer, to middle, to inner ear and is processed through the auditory pathways to the cortex. Thresholds for the right ear are marked by Os and for the left ear by Xs. Traditionally, right and left ear responses were marked in red and blue ink, respectively, but because so many charts are Faxed and photocopied, this practice has become less common. If thresholds are beyond the maximum output limits of the audiometer, a downward pointing arrow is used to indicate the absence of response.

The **pure tone average (PTA)** is commonly used to report the degree of hearing loss. The PTA is the simple average of the air-conduction thresholds at 500, 1000, and 2000 Hz and is computed separately for each ear. The PTA does not reflect the **configuration** or shape of the audiometric pattern. The configuration is usually also described in the report indicating whether the loss is "low frequency," "sloping high frequency," "flat," or of another configuration.

Sound-field testing also uses the air-conduction pathway and is performed through speakers on each side of the patient, usually placed at 45° angles. It is commonly used for infants and young children who cannot be tested under earphones. In **Visual reinforcement audiometry (VRA) or Conditioned orientation response audiometry (COR)**, whenever a child turns his or her head toward the sound source just after a signal is presented, a toy is illuminated and/or animated. If the child turns toward the speaker when there is no signal, no reinforcement is provided.

Generally, thresholds can be obtained and they are marked as wavy lines on the audiogram. Sound-field testing does not provide separate threshold information for each ear, but rather thresholds will reflect hearing in the better ear. If the child can quickly and consistently localize the sound source however, she or he probably has balanced hearing between the two ears. Asymmetric hearing thresholds will impair sound localization.

Sometimes, sound-field testing is used to measure **functional gain** in hearing aids. Functional gain is the difference between a patient's sound-field thresholds with and without the hearing aids. Each "aided" threshold is generally marked by "A."

While air-conduction and sound-field testing deliver signals through the air, bone-conduction testing delivers signals through a small vibrator usually placed on the mastoid or forehead. The signal is conducted to the cochlea through the skull, thus bypassing the outer and middle ear. Bone-conduction thresholds are indicated by a "<" for the right ear and a ">" for the left ear. Sometimes, for high (35–50 dB HL) intensities at the low frequencies of 250 Hz or 500 Hz the patient may feel rather than hear the signal. This response is called a **vibrotactile response** and does not reflect actual hearing. Such a response would be indicated by a "VT" on the audiogram.

An **air-bone gap** occurs when the bone-conduction threshold is 10 dB better than the air-conduction threshold for a given frequency. An air-bone gap suggests a conductive problem resulting from abnormality in the outer or middle ear. When air- and bone-conduction thresholds are the same, no conductive hearing loss is indicated. Types of hearing loss are discussed later in this chapter.

Air- and bone-conduction testing may be called **pure-tone testing** because tones containing a single frequency are used as stimuli. Sound-field testing requires that "warble tones" or "narrow bands of noise" be used as stimuli. When a pure-tone signal bounces back in a sound field, the reflected signal may interfere with the original signal being delivered. Small holes manufactured in sound booth walls reduce but do not eliminate this problem.

Usually, an audiogram will also have an indication of **reliability**. An audiologist will usually repeat threshold testing at one or more frequencies to determine the reliability of threshold determination for that patient. A cooperative, attentive patient should yield thresholds that are replicable within 5 dB. Reliability within 5 dB is listed as "good," within 10 dB as "fair," and worse than 10 dB as "poor." Fair or poor reliability suggests that the patient either did not understand or did not cooperate for the test.

MASKING

Sometimes a noise is presented to the nontest ear to prevent it from responding to a signal presented to the test ear. This noise is called **masking** and the resultant thresholds in the test ear, which should then represent actual threshold for the test ear, are called **masked thresholds.** On the audiogram, masked air-conduction thresholds are indicated by triangles (Δ) for the right ear and squares (□) for the left ear. Masked bone-conduction thresholds are marked by "[" for the right ear and "]" for the left ear. (Fig 1-1).

Interaural attenuation is the amount a signal is reduced in traveling from the test to the nontest ear. For air-conducted signals delivered

SYMBOLS		
	Right	Left
Air Unmasked	O	X
Air Masked	Δ	□
Bone Unmasked	<	>
Bone Masked	[	]
Sound Field	S	S
Aided	A	A

Fig 1. — The symbols typically used on audiograms.

through a standard earphone, interaural attenuation is approximately 40 dB although it may be somewhat less for low frequencies and more for the higher frequencies. For bone conduction, the interaural attenuation may be 0 dB because bone conducts sound very effectively. Therefore, masking is more frequently used in bone-conduction testing. Unmasked bone-conduction thresholds will reflect the threshold of the better ear, not necessarily the intended test ear.

Masking is needed whenever the signal presented to the test ear could possibly be detected by the nontest ear more readily than the test ear. For air-conduction testing, this generally occurs when the bone-conduction threshold (not the air-conduction threshold) of the nontest ear is 40 dB better than the unmasked air-conduction threshold in the test ear because the signal would not be sufficiently reduced by interaural attenuation before reaching the nontest ear. A shadow curve can occur in this situation. A **shadow curve** is obtained when the thresholds recorded for the test ear actually reflect the responses of the cochlea of the nontest ear. In this case, even a totally deaf ear will appear to have responses only 40 dB or so worse than the bone-conduction thresholds of the nontest ear. Appropriate masking will eliminate the shadow curve and reveal the true responses for the test ear.

In bone-conduction testing, masking is generally used whenever there is an air-bone gap. Because interaural attenuation for bone conduction is close to 0 dB, a marked asymmetry in bone conduction between the two ears is not necessary for contralateralization of the response to occur.

A **masking dilemma** occurs when the masking presented to the nontest ear can cross over to the test ear and interfere with the test ear's threshold measurement. Usually a masking dilemma occurs when a patient has a large bilateral conductive hearing loss. For example, if the patient has an air-conduction threshold in the test ear of 60 dB and a bone-conduction threshold in the nontest ear of 0 dB, the signal presented to the test ear would be detected in the nontest ear at approximately 20 dB above threshold. However, if the nontest ear also has a 60 dB conductive hearing loss, masking noise would then be delivered to the nontest ear at a minimum of 70 dB HL which, after approximately 40 dB interaural attenuation, would arrive at the test ear at approximately 30 dB. If the bone-conduction threshold of the test ear is also 0 dB, the masking noise would mask not only the nontest ear but the test ear as well. Insert earphones, which provide greater interaural attenuation, and other test techniques may be helpful but nonetheless masking dilemmas can be problematic.

Simply placing an earphone over the nontest ear may falsely improve a bone-conduction threshold because of the **occlusion effect**. The phenomenon can be demonstrated by simply humming at a low frequency and then occluding one ear. Immediately, the low-frequency signal sounds louder in the occluded ear. Therefore, bone conduction is usually tested first without a contralateral earphone in place and an earphone is placed only if masking is required. If unmasked bone-conduction thresholds suggest an air-bone gap and masked thresholds show no air-bone gap in either ear, the unmasked bone conduction thresholds may have been falsely improved by the presence of an earphone. Typically the occlusion effect is observed only at the test frequencies of 250 Hz to 1000 Hz. The effect decreases as test frequency increases.

SPEECH TESTING

Although commonly called "speech tests," speech testing in audiology does not assess the patient's speech, but rather his or her ability to perceive and recognize speech and speech signals. Numerous tests exist for testing speech perception including very sophisticated tests for special applications. However, the basic audiologic assessment generally includes the **speech reception threshold (SRT)** and **word recognition** measures. Sometimes "word recognition" is referred to as "speech discrimination," particularly in older texts.

Speech reception threshold measures the lowest intensity level at which the patient can correctly repeat 50% of common bisyllabic words like "hotdog" or "baseball" which are delivered with equal emphasis on both syllables. The SRT threshold should closely correspond to the audiogram PTA. If the SRT is substantially better than the PTA, the patient may be feigning or exaggerating a hearing loss. If the SRT is poorer than the PTA, the patient may have a hearing loss that severely distorts speech. In either case, the patient may not have understood the directions and should be reinstructed before further testing. When a patient has difficulty understanding speech, or is hesitant to guess, a **"limited set"** of SRT test words may be used. In this case, the audiologist may practice a set of approximately six words with the patient and then use only those familiar words in testing. For a limited set of SRT words, SRT threshold may more closely approximate threshold of the best frequency used to compute the PTA rather than the PTA itself. Toddlers may simply be asked to point to various facial parts ("Point to your nose") to obtain the SRT.

Speech detection threshold (SDT) measures the lowest intensity level at which the patient can detect the presence of speech, not necessarily bisyllabic words. It is used when an SRT cannot be obtained. For example, an infant cannot repeat words but can be conditioned to respond to the presence of speech in the same manner as for other types of stimuli discussed above. SDT generally will correspond to the threshold of the best test frequency threshold.

Speech discrimination or **word recognition** measures the patient's ability to repeat a list of single syllable words at a suprathreshold level approximately 40 dB above the SRT or at a comfortable listening level if 40 dB is too loud for the patient. The test level used may be indicated in HL or in **sensation level (SL)**. Sensation level is simply the difference between the patient's threshold for a given signal and the actual presentation level of the same signal.

Traditionally, these tests have been called "speech discrimination" tests, but the term "word recognition" is becoming more commonly used because it more accurately reflects the patient's task. The premise is to measure how well a patient understands speech when it is comfortably loud enough.

Several tests exist, including those that emphasize consonants, but the most commonly used test employs **phonetically balanced (PB)** word lists. These word lists contain phonemes with the same frequency that they typically occur in the test language. Scores are presented as the percentage of words correctly repeated from lists of 50 or 25 words. Some hearing losses, even when of a mild degree, can cause very poor speech discrimination, whereas other losses of a greater degree may not greatly distort speech signals. However, some correspondence between the audiometric pattern and/or etiology of the hearing loss is expected.

Performance intensity functions (PI functions or PIPB functions) consist of testing word recognition (as described above) at several different intensity levels. This test can serve several purposes. From the PI function the **PB max**, or the intensity level providing the best word recognition score, can be determined. The PB max can be helpful in setting the gain for a hearing aid or in selecting the optimal level for other tests. The PI function can also be used as a site of lesion test by determining if **rollover**, a worsening of the word recognition score, occurs at high intensities. In conductive or cochlear loss, word recognition scores should continue to improve or remain the same as stimulus intensity increases. In retrocochlear lesions, as in the case of an acoustic neuroma, scores may reach PB max and then deteriorate.

Many other types of tests use speech or speechlike stimuli. These stimuli may include nonsense syllables, sentences, numbers, synthetically derived (computer-generated) speech signals, or altered (e.g., time-compressed or filtered) speech signals. However, the most commonly used tests are those described above.

THE BASIC BATTERY

Sometimes the term **"basic battery"** is used to describe the combination of tests including pure tone air- and bone-conduction thresholds, SRT, and word recognition. Some audiologists include immittance audiometry (described in a separate chapter) in their "basic battery."

Abbreviations Used in Reports

CNT Could not test

DNT Did not test

HA Hearing aid

HAE Hearing aid evaluation (discussed in chapter on hearing aids but listed here because it is frequently listed in the recommendations)

HFHL High-frequency hearing loss

NR No response

SNHL Sensorineural hearing loss

VT Vibrotactile response

WNL Within normal limits

TYPES OF HEARING LOSS

Conductive Hearing Loss

If bone-conduction thresholds are substantially better than air-conduction thresholds, the patient has a **conductive hearing loss**, suggesting that an abnormality in the outer or middle ear is causing the hearing loss. Typically, conductive hearing losses have a fairly flat (equal loss at all test frequencies) configuration but exceptions exist. Most conductive hearing losses are of a slight to mild degree. Even a **maximal conductive hearing loss** does not exceed 60–70 dB HL because, even with no outer or middle ear, sound at 60 to 70 dB HL will stimulate the cochlea directly. Therefore, a patient cannot have a profound hearing loss with no sensorineural component.

Usually conductive hearing losses only cause a loss of intensity with little or no signal distortion. Therefore, word recognition is usually normal at an adequate sensation level.

The most common causes of conductive hearing loss include cerumen or foreign body occlusion of the ear canal, tympanic membrane perforation, otitis media, or other middle ear growth or abnormality, either acquired or congenital. Most conductive hearing losses can be treated medically and/or surgically, but when they cannot be corrected, these patients do very well with hearing aids because of their excellent speech discrimination.

Sensorineural Hearing Loss

If air- and bone-conduction thresholds are equal, but poorer than normal, the patient has a **sensorineural hearing loss**. Theoretically, the loss would be sensory if only the cochlea was involved and neural if the loss was purely retrocochlear, but in clinical practice it is frequently difficult to distinguish clearly between sensory and neural components, and some disorders (e.g., presbycusis, acoustic neuromas, etc.) may have both sensory and neural components. Therefore, the term "sensorineural" is commonly used. Typically the sensorineural hearing loss is sloping, sometimes precipitously, with poorer hearing for the higher frequencies. Consequently, the patient may hear the vowels (that have primarily low-frequency content) better than the consonants (that have primarily high-frequency content) so "they can hear but they cannot understand" speech. High-frequency voices, such as children's, may be particularly difficult for them to understand. Patients with sensorineural hearing loss have particular trouble understanding speech in background noise.

Shouting generally is not helpful because shouting primarily increases the intensity level of the vowels rather than the consonants. Shouting often violates the patient's comfort levels without improving speech understanding. Also, sensorineural hearing loss tends to be associated with **recruitment**. Recruitment is an abnormal increase in the loudness of sound. Therefore, these patients cannot hear soft sounds but a small or moderate increase in sound intensity is perceived as a large growth in loudness. Intense sounds may be more painful for these patients than for the normally hearing person. These patients are then said to have a **limited dynamic range**. In other words, the range of usable hearing between threshold and an **uncomfortable loudness level** (UCL) (UCL – threshold = dynamic range) is abnormally small.

Patients with sensorineural hearing loss can usually be fitted with hearing aids, or cochlear implants for profound loss, but hearing is generally not restored to normal. When cochlear hair cells and/or neurons are missing, the ear will distort whatever sound is presented to the ear. Great advances in hearing aids have been made, but no hearing aid can totally compensate for the damaged auditory system.

Most sensorineural hearing losses do not respond to medical and/or surgical treatment.

In many cases, the exact etiology of a sensorineural hearing loss cannot be precisely determined and causal factors may be cumulative over a lifetime. However, common causes include noise exposure; aging; familial hearing loss; Ménière's disease; infections including measles, mumps, meningitis, cytomegalovirus (in utero); low birth weight; and a number of genetic syndromes.

Mixed hearing loss is simply a combination of both sensorineural and conductive hearing loss.

The terms **functional hearing loss, pseudohypacusis,** or **nonorganic hearing loss** mean that the loss is feigned or exaggerated. Functional hearing loss generally is characterized by poor reliability, poor agreement between SRT and PTA, and atypical speech discrimination errors.

DEGREES OF HEARING LOSS

Degrees of hearing loss are formally based on the PTA for each ear. Because the degree alone does not specify configuration, sometimes the report will specify degree of loss for each frequency region. For example, the patient's hearing loss may be described as "mild for the low and mid frequencies and severe for the high frequencies." However, if the loss is simply categorized as "moderate," that categorization is based on the PTA (Fig 1–2).

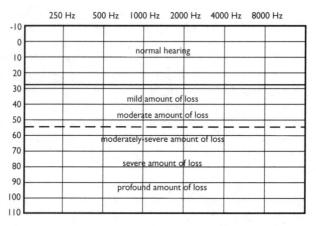

Fig 1-2. — The degree of hearing loss (as computed on the basis of PTA).

The following categories are from Goodman 1965 using American National Standards Institute (ANSI) or International Standards Organization (ISO) references for signal intensity. From 1951 to 1964, American Standards Association (ASA) references were used and audiograms obtained from those times will have to be converted accordingly.

ANSI	Degree of Loss
−10 to 26 dB	Within normal limits
27 to 40 dB	Mild loss
41 to 55 dB	Moderate loss
56 to 70 dB	Moderately severe loss
71 to 90 dB	Severe loss
91+ dB	Profound loss

Note that thresholds sometimes will be listed as "borderline normal" if they are at 25 dB; or if air-bone gaps are present but air-conduction thresholds are technically within normal limits, the thresholds may be described as a "slight conductive hearing loss."

Summary: The basic audiologic assessment can yield a great deal of information about a patient's hearing including the type and degree of hearing loss, the impact of the hearing loss on word recognition ability and the reliabilty of the measures for a given patient.

Self-Assessment Questions

(Answers and Explanations Follow)

1. What is the difference between dB SPL and dB HL?

2. What is the PTA for the right ear in the following audiogram?

FREQUENCY IN HERTZ (Hz)

	Right	Left
SYMBOLS		
	Right	Left
Air Unmasked	O	X
Air Masked	Δ	□
Bone Unmasked	<	>
Bone Masked	[	]
Sound Field	S	S
Aided	A	A

RELIABILITY: ☑ GOOD   ☐ FAIR   ☐ POOR

SPEECH AUDIOMETRY

	SPEECH RECEPTION THRESHOLD	SPEECH DETECTION THRESHOLD	MASK	WORD RECOGNITION - QUIET					
				%	HL	MASK	%	HL	MASK
R	35			20%	75	✓	%		
L	0			100%	40	✓	%		
SF									

3. The following audiogram shows a _____(type) hearing loss of a _____(degree) in the right ear and a _____(type) hearing loss of a _____(degree) in the left ear.

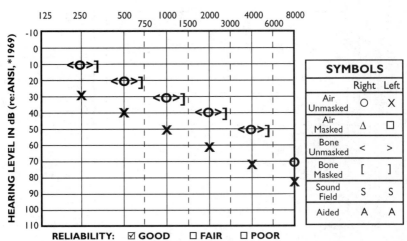

FREQUENCY IN HERTZ (Hz)

SYMBOLS		
	Right	Left
Air Unmasked	O	X
Air Masked	Δ	□
Bone Unmasked	<	>
Bone Masked	[	]
Sound Field	S	S
Aided	A	A

RELIABILITY: ☑ **GOOD**   □ **FAIR**   □ **POOR**

SPEECH AUDIOMETRY								
	SPEECH RECEPTION THRESHOLD	SPEECH DETECTION THRESHOLD	MASK	WORD RECOGNITION - QUIET					
				%	HL	MASK	%	HL	MASK
R	30			86%	70	✓	%		
L	45			82%	85	✓	%		
SF									

4. The following is an example of a _____.

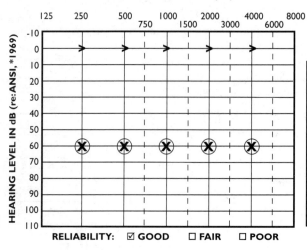

FREQUENCY IN HERTZ (Hz)

RELIABILITY: ☑ GOOD   ☐ FAIR   ☐ POOR

SYMBOLS		
	Right	Left
Air Unmasked	O	X
Air Masked	Δ	☐
Bone Unmasked	<	>
Bone Masked	[	]
Sound Field	S	S
Aided	A	A

5. The following is an example of a _____.

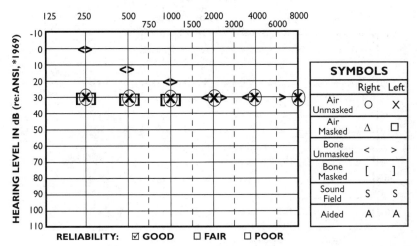

FREQUENCY IN HERTZ (Hz)

SYMBOLS		
	Right	Left
Air Unmasked	O	X
Air Masked	Δ	□
Bone Unmasked	<	>
Bone Masked	[	]
Sound Field	S	S
Aided	A	A

RELIABILITY: ☑ GOOD ☐ FAIR ☐ POOR

SPEECH AUDIOMETRY									
	SPEECH RECEPTION THRESHOLD	SPEECH DETECTION THRESHOLD	MASK	WORD RECOGNITION - QUIET					
				%	HL	MASK	%	HL	MASK
R	25			92%	65		%		
L	25			92%	65		%		
SF									

6. The following is an example of _____.

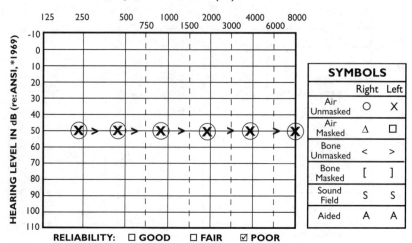

FREQUENCY IN HERTZ (Hz)

SYMBOLS		
	Right	Left
Air Unmasked	O	X
Air Masked	Δ	□
Bone Unmasked	<	>
Bone Masked	[	]
Sound Field	S	S
Aided	A	A

RELIABILITY: □ GOOD   □ FAIR   ☑ POOR

SPEECH AUDIOMETRY									
	SPEECH RECEPTION THRESHOLD	SPEECH DETECTION THRESHOLD	MASK	WORD RECOGNITION - QUIET					
				%	HL	MASK	%	HL	MASK
R	30			50%	70		%		
L	30			32%	70		%		
SF									

7. The following is an example of _____.

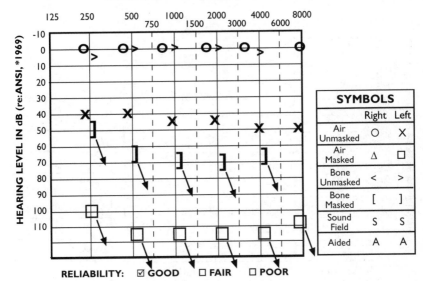

FREQUENCY IN HERTZ (Hz)

SYMBOLS

	Right	Left
Air Unmasked	O	X
Air Masked	Δ	□
Bone Unmasked	<	>
Bone Masked	[	]
Sound Field	S	S
Aided	A	A

RELIABILITY: ☑ **GOOD** □ **FAIR** □ **POOR**

8. In this audiogram the child has a _____(type) hearing

loss of a _____(degree) in _____(which ear).

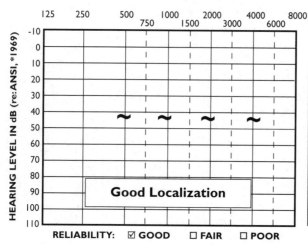

FREQUENCY IN HERTZ (Hz)

SYMBOLS		
	Right	Left
Air Unmasked	O	X
Air Masked	Δ	□
Bone Unmasked	<	>
Bone Masked	[	]
Sound Field	S	S
Aided	A	A

RELIABILITY: ☑ **GOOD**   ☐ **FAIR**   ☐ **POOR**

SPEECH AUDIOMETRY									
	SPEECH RECEPTION THRESHOLD	SPEECH DETECTION THRESHOLD	MASK	WORD RECOGNITION - QUIET					
				%	HL	MASK	%	HL	MASK
R				%			%		
L				%			%		
SF	45			Good Localization					

9. The following audiogram shows a _____ (type) hearing loss

of a _____ (degree) in _____ (which ear).

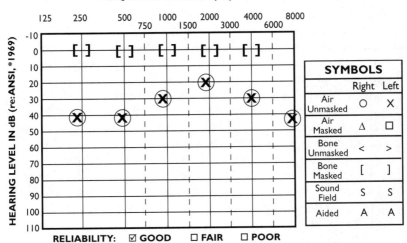

Answers to Self-Assessment Questions

1. HL is referenced to the threshold of normal human hearing at each frequency. SPL is referenced to an absolute sound pressure level. They are related but not equal. Because the ear is nonlinear, less signal intensity in SPL is required for 0 dB HL at the mid frequencies than at the low or high frequencies.

2. The PTA is 40 dB HL. It is the average of the air-conduction thresholds for the right ear at 500, 1000, and 2000 Hz. Note that when masked and unmasked thresholds are given, always use the masked thresholds because they represent actual threshold. Also note that masking was needed for the high frequencies in this case because thresholds were 40 dB poorer in the right ear than in the left ear and the signal contralateralized to the better ear because interaural attenuation for air-conducted signals is approximately 40 dB. Masking was also needed for bone-conduction testing because interaural attenuation for bone-conducted signals can be 0 dB. Without masking this sensorineural hearing loss would have appeared to be conductive.

   A unilateral sensorineural hearing loss like this with very poor speech discrimination could be caused by an acoustic neuroma on the VIIIth nerve.

3. This audiogram shows a sensorineural hearing loss of a mild degree in the right ear and a mixed hearing loss of a moderate degree in the left ear. This audiogram could easily occur in someone with bilateral presbycusis as well as otitis media in the left ear.

4. This is an example of a masking dilemma. An adequate level of masking would have to be at least 70 dB HL at any frequency which would arrive at the opposite cochlea at approximately 30 dB HL. All you know from this audiogram is that at least one ear has normal bone-conduction thresholds and no worse than 60 dB HL air conduction thresholds. However, you can't tell which ear it is. In fact, one ear could be totally deaf.

5. This is an example of the occlusion effect. Note that unmasked bone-conduction thresholds are substantially better than masked bone-conduction thresholds in either ear and this effect is more pronounced as the frequency decreases. There is no true conductive component to this hearing loss. This artifact could have been avoided by testing unmasked bone conduction without the masking earphone on the contralateral ear.

6. This would probably be a functional (feigned or exaggerated) hearing loss. Note that the reliability is poor and the SRTs are substantially better than air-conduction threshold at any of the test frequencies.

7. This is an example of a shadow curve. The left ear appears to have only a moderate hearing loss without masking. However, the responses are entirely due to the signal contralateralizing and being detected in the better ear. With masking, thresholds are beyond the maximum output limits of the audiometer revealing that the ear is actually deaf.

8. This audiogram would usually be obtained for an infant or toddler using COR or VRA. The degree of loss is moderate but you only know that the thresholds are for the better ear. You cannot tell from the audiogram if the ears are different, and if so, which ear is the better ear. However, the good localization noted for both the SDT and the frequency-specific stimuli would suggest balanced hearing. The information is not sufficient to determine the type of hearing loss.

9. This audiogram shows a conductive hearing loss of a mild degree in both ears. This loss can commonly occur in otitis media.

References and Further Reading

1. Arlinger S, ed. *Manual of Practical Audiometry.* London, England: Whurr Publishers Ltd; 1991
2. Goodman A. Reference zero levels, for pure-tone audiometers. *Asha.* 1965; 7:262–263.
3. Hall, JW, Mueller, HG. *Audiologists' Desk Reference.* vol 1. San Diego, Calif: Singular Publishing Group Inc; 1997
4. Katz J, ed. *Handbook of Clinical Audiology.* Baltimore, Md: Williams and Wilkins; 1985
5. Martin, FN, ed. *Medical Audiology: Disorders of Hearing.* Englewood Cliffs, NJ: Prentice-Hall; 1981

2

Immittance Audiometry (Tympanometry and Acoustic Reflexes)

OVERVIEW: This chapter describes immittance audiometry, generally used for assessing tympanic membrane and middle ear function, and acoustic reflexes. Interpretation of results is included.

DESCRIPTION OF THE TESTS

Immittance audiometry measures the function of the tympanic membrane, middle ear, and the acoustic reflex pathway. It does not measure "hearing."

In **immittance audiometry** a soft plastic probe is seated in the outer third of the ear canal. An airtight seal must be obtained but no behavioral response of the patient is required. The patient simply has to sit quietly during the test. Most equipment measures **admittance** or the amount of sound transmitted through the middle ear system. Other systems measure **impedance** or the amount of sound that is not transmitted or is reflected back. The term **immittance** is a more general term that includes either admittance or impedance. Clinically, it makes little difference which term is used because admittance and impedance are reciprocals of each other and the results are essentially equivalent regardless of the actual recording technique used. Several test measures can be obtained.

Tympanometry

For **tympanometry**, a probe tone, usually (but not always) at 220 Hz, is introduced into the ear. The amount of sound reflected back from the tympanic membrane is then measured as the pressure in the ear canal is varied from positive to negative pressure.

The **tympanogram** is a graph that plots the variation in air pressure (measured in **decaPascals** or **daPa**) on the X axis to immittance (measured in **millimhO** or **mmhO for admittance** which is the reciprocal of mOhms for impedance) on the Y axis as air pressure in the ear canal is varied. When the pressure in the ear canal approximates the pressure in the middle ear cavity, a **peak** occurs in the tympanogram because the admittance of the middle ear system is greatest (and thus the impedance is least) when the pressure in the ear canal is matched to the pressure in the middle ear cavity.

In a normal ear, the peak will occur at atmospheric pressure (0) because the Eustachian tube is functioning normally and periodically ventilating the middle ear to keep it at atmospheric pressure. The normal tympanic membrane and middle ear also have normal compliance or mobility. This type of tympanogram is called a Type **A tympanogram** (Fig 2–1). If the Eustachian tube is functioning properly but the tympanic membrane is thickened or scarred or the middle ear system is stiff, such as in otosclerosis or "glue ear," the pressure peak will occur at normal pressure but will be reduced in height which is called a **Type A$_S$ tympanogram** (Fig 2–2) because it is "shallow." If the Eustachian tube is functioning properly but the system is hypermobile,

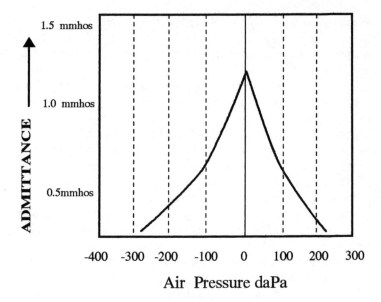

Fig 2-1. — Type A tympanogram showing normal middle ear pressure and compliance.

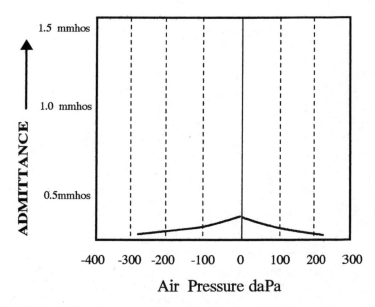

Fig 2-2. — Type A$_S$ tympanogram showing normal middle ear pressure but low compliance.

as in ossicular discontinuity or a flaccid tympanic membrane, the peak will be at or near atmospheric pressure but the peak will be very high or even off the chart, which is called a **Type A$_d$ tympanogram** (Fig 2–3) because it is "deep."

If the middle ear is full of fluid as in otitis media, the air pressure in the ear canal will not match to the fluid-filled middle ear and only a flat trace, called a **Type B tympanogram** (Fig 2–4), will be obtained. A Type B tympanogram will also be obtained if the ear canal or probe is occluded by cerumen or if there is a perforation in the tympanic membrane (TM). In the case of a perforated TM, it is often impossible to obtain a seal because air pressure introduced to the ear canal passes through the middle ear and escapes through the Eustachian tube. The different types of Type B tympanograms can be distinguished from one another on the basis of volume as measured by static compliance and described below.

If the Eustachian tube is not functioning properly as seen in early or resolving otitis media, a negative pressure can develop in the middle ear. Therefore the peak will be at negative pressure which is called a **Type C tympanogram** (Fig 2–5). Sometimes a peak at positive pressure will be obtained in early otitis media. This configuration can be called a **Type P tympanogram** but the designation is rarely used.

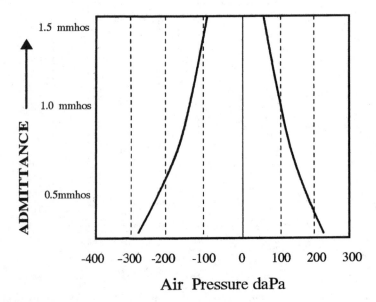

Fig 2-3. — Type A$_d$ tympanogram showing normal middle ear pressure but high compliance.

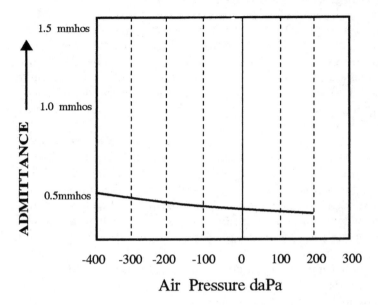

Fig 2-4. — Type B tympanogram with no clear pressure peak, an essentially flat tracing.

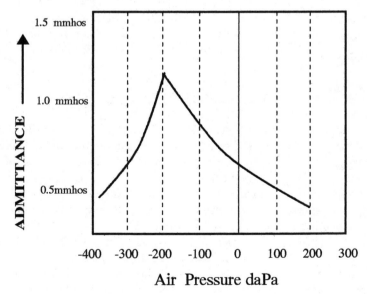

Fig 2-5. — Type C tympanogram showing significant negative pressure.

Additional Clinical Considerations

Tympanometry, using standard protocols, may not be valid on infants below 7 months of age because the cartilage of the ear canal is so soft that the air pressure variations expand and contract the volume of the ear canal giving the false appearance of middle ear compliance changes. Research is currently being conducted in an attempt to establish appropriate protocols and interpretation guidelines for infants below 7 months of age.

A glomus jugulare tumor, a carotid bruit, a patulous Eustachian tube, or palatal myoclonus can cause **oscillations in the tympanogram**. These oscillations can be seen more easily in the acoustic reflex recording mode because the vertical scale is expanded. These disorders can be distinguished from one another because in the glomus jugulare tumor and the carotid artery bruit the rate of oscillation will correspond to the pulse. Pressure on the carotid artery will eliminate the pulsing in the case of a carotid bruit. In the case of a patulous Eustachian tube, the oscillations will correspond to the patient's breathing. Palatal myoclonus will cause very small and fast oscillations, frequently over 100 per minute.

Some individuals use immittance equipment to perform a "fistula test" or to look for "Hennebert's sign." In this procedure, +200 daPa pressure is introduced into the ear canal and maintained for approximately 30 s. (Sometimes alternating presentations of positive and negative pressure epochs are presented.) The patient is then checked for the presence of nystagmus and/or dizziness. If either is present, the findings are considered positive for the presence of perilymphatic fistula. However, the accuracy of this test has been questioned.

STATIC COMPLIANCE

Static compliance is measured at +200 daPa **(C1)** and again at the peak of the tympanogram **(C2)**. C1 provides a volume reading in cubic centimeters (cc). If the ear canal or probe is filled with cerumen or debris, the volume reading will be very low. These problems can then be corrected and another measure can be obtained. If the tympanic membrane is perforated, a high volume reading will be obtained because the probe is measuring the volume of both the ear canal and the middle ear. This indication of a perforation is sometimes used to check the patency of pressure equalization tubes (PE tubes) inserted in the tympanic membrane to treat otitis media. If the volume is normal and a Type B tympanogram is obtained, usually otitis media is the underlying cause. However, whenever a Type B tympanogram is obtained, it is critical to check the volume reading (C1) for differential diagnosis.

The difference between C1 and C2 is **Cx**. Commonly the term **"static compliance"** is used to refer to Cx or the difference between the compliance reading at +200 daPa and at the peak of the tympanogram. Basically this represents the height of the peak on the tympanogram. Thus, a Type A tympanogram would have normal static compliance, a Type B tympanogram would have very low static compliance, and a Type A_d would have very high static compliance.

ACOUSTIC REFLEXES

An acoustic reflex occurs when the stapedius muscle in the middle ear contracts in response to an intense sound. Even when the stimulus is monaural, the contraction in a normal ear is bilateral. Because the contraction stiffens the ossicular chain, the contraction can be read out as a change in the immittance of the middle ear. If the reflex is read out in the stimulated ear, it is called an **uncrossed** or **ipsilateral reflex**. If it is read out in the opposite ear, it is called a **crossed** or **contralateral reflex**. Tympanograms are always obtained before acoustic reflexes because reflexes must be tested with pressure set at the point of maximum compliance or "the peak of the tympanogram."

The **physiologic utility** of acoustic reflexes is controversial. These reflexes do attentuate sound input to the ear but this relatively small effect occurs primarily at low frequencies and fatigues. Therefore, the effect cannot adequately protect against continuous noise exposure. Additionally, the onset of the acoustic reflex may be too slow to adequately protect against impact noise. The acoustic reflex is activated by the patient's own voice and so may serve to reduce the annoyance level of hearing one's voice too loudly.

Usually we test **crossed** and **uncrossed acoustic reflex thresholds**. In this test, signals of various intensities are presented to the ear to determine the least intense signal that can activate the acoustic reflex. Acoustic reflex thresholds in normals generally occur 70–100 dB above the patient's threshold for that frequency. If retrocochlear lesion is suspected, we may test **acoustic reflex decay**. In this test, a signal 10 dB above the patient's acoustic reflex threshold at either 500 Hz or 1000 Hz is presented to the ear for 10 s and the crossed reflex is monitored. If the amplitude of the response decreases more than 50% during the 10 s interval, it is considered abnormal and indicative of VIIIth nerve disorder. Frequencies above 1000 Hz are not used for testing acoustic reflex decay because decay at high frequencies occurs even in normal subjects. Reflex decay, however, is neither as sensitive nor as specific as the auditory brainstem response (ABR) for detecting acoustic neuromas.

To interpret acoustic reflexes, it is important to know the **anatomy of the ipsilateral** and **contralateral acoustic reflex pathways**. When an intense acoustic signal is presented to the ear, it activates the reflex pathway. This pathway travels up the cochlear branch of the VIIIth nerve of the stimulated ear to the ipsilateral ventral cochlear nucleus through the trapezoid body. Most of the fibers in the ipsilateral pathway then course to the medial part of the ipsilateral facial motor nucleus to the ipsilateral facial nerve and the ipsilateral stapedius muscle. However, some fibers in the ipsilateral pathway course from the trapezoid body to the ipsilateral medial superior olivary complex before coursing to the ipsilateral facial motor nucleus to activate the ipsilateral stapedius muscle contraction. The contralateral pathway similarly travels up the VIIIth nerve and across the trapezoid body. The fibers then course to the ipsilateral medial superior olive and then across to the contralateral facial motor nucleus to activate the contralateral facial nerve and stapedius muscle. Therefore, the contralateral reflex pathway has four neurons and the ipsilateral pathway has primarily three but some four neuron connections.

Acoustic reflexes can be very useful in differential diagnosis. Naturally, a lesion anywhere along the pathway can disrupt the response, but the pattern of abnormality can help identify the site of lesion.

Disorders Affecting the Acoustic Reflexes

- A **lesion of the VIIIth nerve (eg, acoustic neuroma)** will usually cause the crossed and uncrossed acoustic reflexes to be absent or their thresholds elevated whenever the lesioned side is stimulated. Acoustic reflex decay is frequently present. However, crossed and uncrossed reflexes will be normal when the contralateral ear is stimulated.

- A **brainstem lesion** that affects the reflex pathway will generally not affect the uncrossed acoustic reflexes but may eliminate the crossed acoustic reflexes.

- A **facial nerve lesion (eg, Bell's Palsy)** will eliminate the response on the affected side regardless of which side is stimulated. An absent stapedius tendon, which can occur even in individuals with normal hearing, will yield the same acoustic reflex test results.

- Patients with **up to moderate sensorineural hearing loss** generally will yield crossed and uncrossed acoustic reflex thresholds at approximately the same absolute levels as normals. However, because their pure tone thresholds are elevated, the reflex thresholds are present at reduced sensation levels, due to recruitment. **Severe or profound hearing loss** generally will cause the reflexes to be absent. However, some patients with Ménière's disease will have reflex thresholds as low as 15 to 20 dB SL.

- A **conductive hearing loss** will eliminate a response when recorded from the affected side regardless of which ear is stimulated. Even when the stapedius muscle still contracts, the middle ear abnormality will obscure the response. An air-bone gap exceeding 30 dB will also eliminate the response whenever the affected side is stimulated. With smaller air-bone gaps, the stimulus may simply be attenuated by the conductive loss, resulting in elevated but not absent crossed reflexes if recorded out in a normal contralateral ear. Therefore, patients with **bilateral conductive hearing loss** will almost always have absent acoustic reflexes bilaterally for both crossed and uncrossed measures. Patients with **unilateral conductive hearing losses** will have absent uncrossed reflexes and absent or elevated crossed reflexes (depending on the size of the air-bone gap) when the affected side is stimulated. When the normal side is stimulated, the uncrossed reflex thresholds will be normal, but the crossed reflex will be absent because of the absence of response on the affected side.

- **Otosclerosis** will usually cause the reflexes to be absent, as in any other conductive hearing loss. Occasionally, particularly in early otosclerosis, a biphasic acoustic reflex pattern is seen rather than a simple monophasic contraction. Some consider this finding to be pathognomonic for otosclerosis.

- Any type of **muscle disorder** that affects the stapedius muscle **(eg, myasthenia gravis)** can eliminate the acoustic reflexes or cause reflex decay.

- Any **central nervous system depressant, including alcohol**, can depress the amplitude of the response. Because the presence of the response is based on amplitude criteria, the response may be determined to be elevated or absent.

Other Applications of Acoustic Reflexes

The acoustic reflex threshold may be helpful in **setting the maximum power output of hearing aids** when the patient (eg, young child) cannot report when a sound is too loud.

Acoustic reflexes can be helpful in **identifying functional hearing loss.** Feigned severe or profound hearing loss can be easily identified as such when acoustic reflexes are normal and within 15 dB of reported behavioral thresholds in the absence of Ménière's disease.

Sensitivity Prediction with the Acoustic Reflex **(SPAR)** is a test to estimate hearing thresholds on the basis of the difference in acoustic reflex thresholds for pure tone signals and broad bands of noise. Much better methods of assessing hearing in patients who cannot or will not respond are now available, and this test is no longer widely used.

Summary: Immittance audiometry includes tympanometry and acoustic reflex testing. Tympanometry provides quick and reliable information regarding tympanic membrane and middle ear function. Acoustic reflex testing can be used to obtain information regarding VIIth nerve, VIIIth nerve, and brainstem function and can yield valuable information for corroborating threshold information, and fitting hearing aids.

Self-Assessment Questions

1. A patient presents a flat 85 dB HL sensorineural hearing loss bilaterally. Type A tympanograms are present bilaterally. Acoustic reflex thresholds are 95 dB HL at 1000 Hz. What is your diagnosis?

2. A patient has 25 dB HL pure-tone air-conduction thresholds across the frequency range with significant air-bone gaps. Immittance audiometry shows Type A_S tympanograms bilaterally. Acoustic reflex thresholds are slightly elevated and show a curious biphasic pattern. What is the most likely diagnosis?

3. A child has a mild conductive hearing loss with Type B tympanograms bilaterally and absent acoustic reflexes. What essential piece of information is missing?

4. A patient has normal hearing bilaterally with Type A tympanograms. When the right ear is stimulated, the uncrossed reflex threshold is present at 85 dB HL, but the crossed acoustic reflex is absent. When the left ear is stimulated, the crossed reflex is present at 85 dB HL, but the uncrossed reflex is absent. What is your diagnosis?

5. A patient has normal hearing in the left ear but a mild sensorineural hearing loss in the right ear. Tympanometry reveals Type A tympanograms bilaterally. When the left ear is stimulated, crossed and uncrossed acoustic reflexes are present at 80 dB HL, but when the right ear is stimulated, both crossed and uncrossed acoustic reflexes are absent. What is your diagnosis?

6. Following a motor vehicle accident, a patient has a Type B tympanogram with very high volume on the right side and a Type A_d tympanogram on the left side. In fact, the peak of the tympanogram on the left side is off the top of the chart. Because the patient is comatose, no behavioral threshold information is available. What is your diagnosis?

7. A patient with normal hearing and Type A tympanograms bilaterally has normal uncrossed reflexes but absent crossed acoustic reflexes bilaterally. What could account for these findings?

Answers to Self-Assessment Questions

1. This patient is feigning or exaggerating the hearing loss. Acoustic reflex thresholds are only 10 dB above the reported pure-tone behavioral thresholds which is a clear sign of functional hearing loss.

2. These are classic findings for early otosclerosis.

3. The volume measurement (C1) is essential in interpreting type B tympanograms. If the volume reading is very low, the probe could have been merely plugged with cerumen or against the ear canal giving a false reading. If the volume reading is very high, the child could have perforated tympanic membranes or functioning PE tubes. If the volume reading is normal, the child probably has fluid in the middle ears.

4. The problem is clearly on the efferent pathway on the left side. Either facial nerve paralysis or an absent stapedius muscle could account for these findings. However, there is no indication of problems elsewhere in the pathway.

5. The problem appears to be on the VIIIth nerve of the right ear. These are classic findings for an acoustic neuroma.

6. On the left side, there is probably ossicular discontinuity. On the right side, there is a perforation of the tympanic membrane. Ossicular discontinuity or other problems on the right side cannot be ruled out because, no other information can be obtained from tympanometry if there is a perforation of the tympanic membrane.

7. These findings are classic for a brainstem lesion.

References and Further Reading

1. Feldman AS, Wilber LA. *Acoustic Impedance and Admittance—The Measurement of Middle Ear Function.* Baltimore, Md: Williams and Wilkins; 1976.
2. Hall JW, Mueller HG. "Immittance Measurements" In: *Audiologists' Desk Reference.* vol 1. San Diego, Calif: Singular Publishing Group Inc; 1997: 175–234.
3. Katz J. *Handbook of Clinical Audiology.* Baltimore, Md: Williams and Wilkins; 1989.
4. Moller A. *Auditory Physiology.* New York, NY: Academic Press; 1983.
5. Silman S, Silverman C. Acoustic immittance. In: S Gerber, ed. *The Handbook of Pediatric Audiology.* Washington, DC: Galludet University Press; 1996.
6. Van Camp KJ, Margolis RH, Wilson RH, Creten WL, Shanks JE. *Principles of Tympanometry.* Rockville, Md: American Speech-Language Hearing Assn; 1986:24 *ASHA Monographs*

3

Pediatric Audiology

OVERVIEW: This chapter describes referral indications and various methods of testing hearing in children including behavioral observation audiometry, visual response audiometry or conditioned orientation response audiometry, and play audiometry. Screening techniques, particularly for newborns and school-age children, are also discussed. Immittance audiometry, auditory brainstem response testing, and otoacoustic emissions are referred to but are more fully discussed in separate chapters dedicated to them. However, a very brief description of each of these procedures is provided.

First, a brief review of some tests used in pediatric audiology. These tests are more fully discussed in Chapters 2, 4, and 5.

AUDITORY BRAINSTEM RESPONSE (ABR)

The ABR is performed by placing electrodes on the surface of the patient's head and recording the electrical activity of the auditory system, from the VIIIth nerve to the inferior colliculus, in response to acoustic stimuli. The response is read as a series of waveforms. The ABR is used for both hearing screening and testing and to assess the neurologic status of the auditory pathway. The ABR may be absent or its threshold elevated as a result of either peripheral hearing loss or neurologic dysfunction affecting the auditory pathway. (See Chapter 5.)

OTOACOUSTIC EMISSIONS (OAES)

OAEs are tested by sealing a small noninvasive probe in the ear canal and recording sounds that are generated by the cochlea. Some people, usually with normal hearing, have spontaneous otoacoustic emissions (SOAEs), meaning the emissions occur even in the absence of an acoustic stimulus. Because many normally hearing individuals do not have SOAEs, they are not generally used for either screening or testing hearing. Transient evoked otoacoustic emissions (TEOAEs) are sounds generated by the cochlea in response to transient (short duration) acoustic stimuli. Distortion product otoacoustic emissions (DPOAEs) are sounds generated by the cochlea in response to two stimuli delivered to the ear simultaneously. The cochlea then produces another sound (or two) of a different frequency than either of the signals delivered to the ear. Both TEOAEs and DPOAEs are used for hearing screening and testing. TEOAEs may be absent or otherwise abnormal as a result of conductive hearing loss, which can prevent the response from being transmitted from the cochlea back out to the ear canal, or of cochlear dysfunction. However, TEOAEs and DPOAEs are not affected by neurologic dysfunction. (See Chapter 4.)

IMMITTANCE AUDIOMETRY

Immittance audiometry includes tympanometry and acoustic reflex testing. Tympanometry is performed by sealing a small noninvasive probe in the ear canal and presenting a pure-tone signal while varying the air pressure in the ear canal. Tympanometry provides excellent information about the status of the tympanic membrane and middle ear, although it is not a test of hearing. Acoustic reflexes are also performed by sealing the same probe in the ear canal. Acoustic reflexes are elicited in response to high-intensity signals. Because the acoustic reflex arcs involve the cochlear branch of the VIIIth nerve, the ventral cochlear nucleus, the trapezoid body, the medial superior olive, the facial motor nucleus, the facial nerve, and the stapedius muscle, acoustic reflexes can be useful in detecting lesions along those pathways. Additionally, acoustic reflexes can be affected by both conductive and sensorineural hearing loss. Therefore, acoustic reflexes and tympanometry are very useful in site of lesion testing. Although neither tympanometry nor acoustic reflex testing is an actual measure of hearing, they are routinely used in children because of the very high incidence of otitis media in children (over 90% of children will have had otitis media by age 6 years) and because middle ear function must be known to evaluate other tests such as OAEs accurately. Immittance audiometry is commonly used in pediatric testing batteries and sometimes in conjunction with hearing screening. (See Chapter 2.)

HEARING SCREENING VERSUS HEARING TESTING

It is important to distinguish between hearing screening and hearing testing. Hearing screening provides only a pass/fail score that selects individuals who need hearing testing. Hearing testing provides information about the degree and type of hearing loss. First, the types of hearing screenings are described by the child's age followed by the types of hearing tests appropriate for each age group. Tuning fork tests are not discussed because they are not appropriate for accurately screening or testing children's hearing.

Hearing Screening

Newborn Screening

Many, but not all, states require hearing screening in newborns. Because hearing loss at birth is one of the most common (if not the most common) birth defects, screening of infants is advisable. Depending on the study, significant hearing loss at birth occurs in 1.5 to 6 infants out of every 1,000 live births. Normal hearing is critical for speech and language development even in the first few months of life.

Because behavioral measures in newborns are unreliable, the recommended methods are the **auditory brainstem response (ABR)** and/or **otoacoustic emissions (OAEs)**. Currently, extensive research is being conducted to determine if ABRs, OAEs, or some combination of the two measures will yield the highest sensitivity and specificity in diagnosing sensorineural hearing loss at birth. One of the confounding factors is the high incidence of conductive hearing loss secondary to either debris in the ear canal or fluid in the middle ears of newborns. Newborns also are being discharged from hospitals shortly after birth allowing little time for hearing screening or resolution of conductive disorders. Some recommendations suggest screening hearing only of infants in the neonatal intensive care unit where the incidence of hearing loss is highest and the stay is longer. For children who fail the newborn screening, generally testing and possible fitting of hearing aids are recommended when they are 2 months of age. At that time, reliable ABR thresholds can be obtained. Hearing aid fitting is recommended at the earliest possible age to stimulate speech and language development, bonding with the parents, and quite possibly development of the central auditory pathways.

The **ALGO** is an automated ABR screener. It basically records the ABR using click stimuli at 35 dB nHL (see Chapter 5). However, rather than have the tester read and interpret the waveforms, the machine simply compares the results obtained to a template of expected waveforms and scores the results as pass or fail. **The Algo II**, a later version of the device, operates in the same manner but also has a higher intensity stimulus option in addition to the 35 dB nHL stimulation.

The **Crib-O-Gram** used to be helpful in screening infant hearing but has been supplanted by better methods such as ABR and OAEs. The Crib-O-Gram consists of a motion transducer, which is placed under the infant, and an intense sound source. The Crib-O-Gram would present the intense sound stimulus and then measure if a change in the child's movements occurred.

For many years the **High Risk Hearing Register (HRHR)** was used to identify children at risk of hearing loss and identify those who needed to be followed for possible hearing loss. Although risk factors are still considered, the HRHR identifies only approximately half of children with congenital hearing impairment.

This HRHR list has now been expanded to include not only newborns but three different age groups as follows (ASHA 1994):

A. For use in neonates (birth through age 28 days) when universal screening is not available.
  1. Family history of hereditary childhood sensorineural hearing loss.
  2. In utero infection, such as cytomegalovirus, rubella, syphilis, herpes, and toxoplasmosis,
  3. Craniofacial anomalies, including those with morphologic abnormalities of the pinna and ear canal.

4. Birthweight less than 1,500 grams (3.3 lbs).
5. Hyperbilirubinemia at a serum level requiring exchange transfusion.
6. Ototoxic medications, including but not limited to the aminoglycosides, used in multiple courses or in combination with loop diuretics.
7. Bacterial meningitis.
8. Apgar score of 0-4 at 1 minute or 0-6 at 5 minutes.
9. Mechanical ventilation lasting 5 days or longer.
10. Stigmata or other findings associated with a syndrome known to include a sensorineural and/or conductive hearing loss.

B. For use with infants (age 29 days through 2 years) when certain health conditions develop that require rescreening.
1. Parent/caregiver concern regarding hearing, speech, language, and/or developmental delay.
2. Bacterial meningitis and other infections associated with sensorineural hearing loss.
3. Head trauma associated with loss of consciousness or skull fracture.
4. Stigmata or other findings associated with a syndrome known to include a sensorineural and/or conductive hearing loss.
5. Ototoxic medications, including but not limited to chemotherapeutic agents or aminoglycosides, used in multiple courses or in combination with loop diuretics.
6. Recurrent or persistent otitis media with effusion for at least 3 months.

C. For use with infants (age 29 days through 3 years) who require periodic monitoring of hearing.
Some newborns and infants may pass initial hearing screening but require periodic monitoring of hearing to detect delayed-onset sensorineural and/or conductive hearing loss. Infants with these indicators require hearing evaluation at least every 6 months until age 3 years, and at appropriate intervals thereafter.

Indicators associated with delayed onset sensorineural hearing loss include:
1. Family history of hereditary childhood hearing loss.
2. In utero infection, such as cytomegalovirus, rubella, syphilis, herpes, or toxoplasmosis.
3. Neurofibromatosis Type II and neurodegenerative disorders.

Indicators associated with conductive hearing loss include:
1. Recurrent or persistent otitis media with effusion.
2. Anatomic deformities and other disorders that affect Eustachian tube function.
3. Neurodegenerative disorders.

Hearing screening for children age 3 years through third grade is recommended by the guidelines of the American Speech-Language-Hearing Association. The child should pass a screening of 20 dB HL for 1000, 2000, and 4000 Hz pure tones in each ear.

Hearing Testing

The following tests are listed according to developmental age rather than chronological age. Developmental age is based on what a normal child of a given chronological age can do. Therefore, a 3-year-old child, who is developmentally delayed and has the development of a normal 2-year-old, would be considered to be at a 2 year developmental age.

Behavioral Observation Audiometry (BOA)

Used primarily for children 0 to 5 months of developmental age, BOA basically consists of presenting a stimulus and observing the infant's response whether it be an eyeblink (auro-palpebral reflex) or a startle response in an awake infant or arousal from sleep in a sleeping infant. An intense stimulus, frequently 90-100 dB HL, is used. Although generally categorized as hearing "tests," at best these procedures should be considered as only a screening and not threshold determination. An intense signal may elicit a strong response even in a child with moderate sensorineural hearing loss because of recruitment. Because children this age do not condition well to sound, the responses quickly habituate and replicability may be problematic. The strong acoustic stimulus may also elicit a crying spell that may preclude further testing. ABRs and OAEs are accurate for testing infants in this age group and are the recommended procedures. Additionally, the latter procedures provide individual ear information. A signal presented in a sound field (through speakers) travels relatively equally to both ears. Therefore, when an infant responds, it cannot be determined if he or she heard the signal in one or both ears.

Visual Reinforcement Audiometry (VRA) or
Conditioned Orientation Response Audiometry (COR)

Used for children 6 to 24 months of developmental age, in these tests, the infant is usually placed facing forward on a parent's or caretaker's lap in a sound booth. Acoustic signals, usually speech, warbled tones, or narrow bands of noise, are presented at moderately intense levels through speakers at 45° angles, horizontally, from the child's face. At 6 months developmental age, an infant will turn his or her head toward an acoustic signal on the horizontal plane. When the infant turns toward the sound, the response is reinforced by lighting and activating an animated toy on top of the speaker. Once the child is conditioned to sound, the intensity of the signals is reduced and thresholds for the various signals can be determined.

Because all signals are presented in a sound field, the thresholds obtained will be for the "better ear" if there is an asymmetry in hearing. However, if the child can readily localize a sound, it is an indication that the hearing between the two ears is balanced. Asymmetric hearing can preclude good sound localization. Therefore, the audiologist's report frequently will indicate the child's localization ability.

Speech detection threshold (SDT) or speech awareness threshold (SAT) can be obtained using VRA. SDT or SAT is simply the lowest intensity level at which the infant responds to a speech stimulus. SDT should correspond to the best threshold for frequency-specific (warbled tone or narrow-band noise) stimuli.

Visually Reinforced Operant Conditioning Audiometry (VROCA)

Used for children 18 months to 3 years developmental age, VROCA is similar to VRA, but instead of turning toward the stimulus, the child pushes a button when the stimulus is perceived. When the response is correct, the toy is activated. This test can be performed with or without earphones.

Tangibly Reinforced Operant Conditioning Audiometry (TROCA)

Used for children 18 months to 3 years of developmental age this procedure is similar to VROCA, but the child receives tangible reinforcement (eg, candy or cereal) when she or he hears a stimulus and responds appropriately. This test is no longer widely used in the United States.

Play Audiometry

Play audiometry may be used for children 2 to 5 years of developmental age. For this testing the child is conditioned to perform a task (eg, drop a block in a bucket) whenever he or she hears a sound. Once the child is conditioned, threshold can be measured. This test is usually performed under earphones so individual ear information can be obtained. Two-year-olds can be a special challenge, requiring frequent changing of tasks and often a combination of VRA, VROCA, and play audiometry.

Speech Testing

Word recognition testing and speech reception threshold testing can be performed in children but some modifications are required. As described in the VRA section, a **speech detection threshold** can be obtained using VRA methods. **Speech reception threshold** in children of 18 to 36 months developmental age can be obtained by instructing the child to point to facial parts (eg, "Point to your nose"). For children 3 to 5 years developmental age, the child can point to spondee words (eg, baseball, hotdog, etc) having equal stress on both syllables on a picture board. This procedure also can be used for older children or adults with speech problems.

Word recognition tests have been developed and normed for children as young as 3 years old. Again picture boards are frequently used in younger children to faciliate cooperation and to avoid contamination of test results by articulation errors. Special tests have also been developed for deaf children being evaluated for cochlear implantation

OAEs AND ABRs

OAEs and ABRs, as described above, can be used at any age. OAEs are rapidly becoming accepted as a part of most pediatric evaluations. OAEs provide individual ear information about cochlear function in a matter of minutes. They do require that the child be relatively quiet but require no other cooperation and can even be performed when the child is asleep. ABRs are generally more time intensive and may require sedation, particularly in toddlers. However, ABRs can provide an excellent estimation of hearing threshold by individual ear and tests further up the auditory pathway than OAEs. Whenever possible, these tests are combined with behavioral measures because neither ABRs nor OAEs test the child's cortical function or ability to perceive and respond to sound.

WHEN TO REFER FOR TESTING

Any child who fails neonatal screening or has a high risk factor should be followed and tested for possible hearing loss. However, high risk factors will identify only about 50% of children born with hearing loss and may not identify adventitious hearing loss secondary to measles, mumps, meningitis, or other disorders. Additionally familial hearing loss, which is frequently recessive, may develop over time. Any time that parents, caregivers, or teachers suspect hearing loss, a child should be tested. Hearing loss can be mistaken for mental retardation because of its impact on speech and language acquisition, cognitive development, and acquisition of academic and social skills.

A child is never too young to be referred for hearing testing. Screening can be performed at birth, and ABR thresholds and OAEs can be tested and hearing aids fitted at 2 months of age. No child is completely "untestable." ABRs, OAEs, and immittance audiometry can be performed even on a comatose patient.

Frequently, in the US, it is approximately 1 year from the time a child is suspected of having hearing loss to the time actual testing is performed, resulting in unnecessary delays in appropriate intervention. Children have a high incidence of otitis media, but it should never be assumed that hearing loss observed is secondary to otitis media. A sensorineural hearing loss may still be present. Any time a child has speech and/or language delays, developmental, or academic delays, or behavioral problems, hearing should be tested because hearing loss may underlie or exacerbate these disorders.

ADDITIONAL CONSIDERATIONS

Children of 5 years or older behavioral age are generally tested in the same manner as adults although special word lists appropriate for their vocabulary may be used for word recognition testing.

Immittance audiometry is part of the standard test battery for virtually all children because of the high incidence of middle ear problems in this population.

Children who feign hearing loss may have other problems requiring attention. Functional hearing loss is frequently a sign of emotional distress.

It is advantageous to have two audiologists or an audiologist and an assistant work together to test children.

Summary: Hearing can be accurately screened in neonates using OAEs and/or ABRs. Risk factors can help identify children with potential hearing loss but over half of children with congenital deafness have no known risk factor. Hearing can be tested and hearing aids fitted by age 2 months using OAE and ABR techniques with more detailed testing protocols and analysis. For children of 6 months developmental age and above a variety of equipment and test techniques are available depending on the level of child's abilities and cooperation.

Self-Assessment Questions

1. In a group of 2-year-old children, using no equipment, how would you select those children who need hearing tests?

2. Which test procedures are appropriate for an 8-month-old child?

3. A 15-month-old child has normal VRA thresholds, but the audiology report says "poor localization." Why could this occur?

4. The mother of a 3-year-old child reports that he does not seem to be responding well to sound and suspects hearing loss. The child had bacterial meningitis a year ago, but hearing was tested prior to hospital discharge and was normal. Speech and language are normal. What do you tell the mother?

5. A 3-month-old infant previously failed the neonatal ALGO hearing screening when she was 2 days old. When do you refer for testing and what type of tests do you refer for?

6. List five risk factors for hearing loss in infants.

Answers to Self-Assessment Questions

1. Any time a child has a speech, language, or other developmental delay; hearing loss is suspected by the parents or caregivers; or there is a risk factor for congenital or acquired hearing loss, the child should be tested.

2. A developmentally normal 8-month-old child can be tested using VRA or COR procedures to obtain thresholds for frequency-specific speech stimuli. Immittance audiometry is also part of the standard battery for children because of the high incidence of middle ear disorders. OAEs are quickly becoming a part of this battery.

   If hearing loss is identified or if the child does not cooperate for VRA or COR, the child will then be tested using ABR to obtain threshold information for each ear separately. OAEs should also be tested to determine cochlear status. Hearing aids would not necessarily be fitted if ABRs are absent but OAEs are normal because the problem is neural and not cochlear. Thus amplification may be inappropriate.

3. Because VRA testing occurs in a sound field, thresholds will reflect hearing in the "better ear" if there is an asymmetry. The child's inability to localize sound suggests a unilateral hearing loss.

4. Any time hearing loss is suspected, hearing should be tested. Bacterial meningitis may cause progressive hearing loss or other factors may have caused hearing loss in the last year. The impact on speech and language development may not be immediately apparent in adventitious hearing loss, particularly in a bright child who may compensate.

5. The child should be referred for ABR threshold testing and for OAEs. Immitance testing is generally not used below 7 months of age. BOA could be performed but ABR and OAE testing is much more accurate. Hearing aids can be fitted at this age.

6. See listing for high risk hearing register to check your anwers.

References and Further Reading

1. American Speech -Language-Hearing Association, Joint Commission on Infant Hearing. 1994 Position Statement. Asha. 1994; 36:38-41
2. Gabbard SA, ed. Hearing in infants. *Sem Hearing*. 1996;16(2).
3. Gerber S. (ed.) (1996) *The Handbook of Pediatric Audiology*. Wsashington, DC: Gallaudet University Press; 1996.
4. Hall JW. Mueller HG. Pediatric audiology., In: *Audiologists' Desk Reference*. vol 1. San Diego, Calif: Singular Publishing Group Inc; 1997: 429-462.
5. McCormick B. *Pediatric Audiology 0–5 Years*. San Diego, Calif: Singular Publishing Group, Inc; 1993.

4

Otoacoustic Emissions (OAEs): SOAEs, TEOAEs, and DPOAEs

OVERVIEW: This chapter reviews spontaneous otoacoustic emissions (SOAEs), transient evoked otoacoustic emissions (TEOAEs), and distortion product otoacoustic emissions (DPOAEs). Emphasis is placed on clinical applications of these techniques. Stimulus frequency otoacoustic emissions (SFOAEs) are only defined because they are not in common clinical use.

THE RESPONSES

Otoacoustic emissions (OAEs) are acoustic signals generated by the cochlea. OAEs can be recorded by a small microphone placed in the ear canal. Although OAEs are relatively easy to record, a good probe fit and noise level control are essential for optimal recording and interpretation because OAEs are very small (usually less than 20 dB SPL).

One of the primary advantages of OAEs is that they are objective, noninvasive responses that are specific to cochlear function. Cochlear outer hair cells are motile (ie, they can expand and contract in response to stimulation). It is widely believed that this outer hair cell motility underlies OAE generation.

Although OAEs are generated in the cochlea, a problem in the outer or middle ear may preclude OAE recording, not only because the presence of a conductive component reduces the stimulation signal intensity but because the signal generated by the cochlea must travel out through the middle and outer ear to be detected by the recording microphone.

SOAEs occur spontaneously (ie, even in the absence of acoustic stimulation). When they occur, they are considered to be a sign of a normally functioning cochlea. However, because they occur in less than half of people with normal hearing, they are not a reliable screening tool (ie, the presence of SOAEs suggests normal cochlear function, but the absence of SOAEs does not necessarily indicate abnormality). SOAEs occur as spikes in the spectrum recorded from the ear canal (Fig 4–1). At first, it was thought that SOAEs might correlate with tinnitus. However, with some exceptions, patients with tinnitus tend not to have SOAEs. Tinnitus frequently occurs with cochlear damage, thus rendering the presence of OAEs less likely. TEOAE generation is preneural and hair cell dependent. However, if a retrocochlear lesion affects the cochlear blood supply, OAEs may be affected.

TEOAEs occur in response to a transient, or short duration signal. Stimuli can be clicks or tone bursts. Usually, click stimuli are employed. Although click stimuli are broad-band signals, the cochlear response can be analyzed to provide frequency-specific information. Currently, only one TEOAE system is available, but other systems will probably be developed in the late 1990s when the patent on the current system expires. In the current system, alternate responses to stimulation are stored in either memory bank A or B. The cross correlation between the averaged recordings in the two memory banks indicates the replicable response component. Generally, a cross correlation exceeding either 50% or 70%, depending on the lab standards, is used to indicate the presence of a response. However, the cross correlation by octave band is more important than the overall correlation because it provides more frequency-specific information. In the time domain,

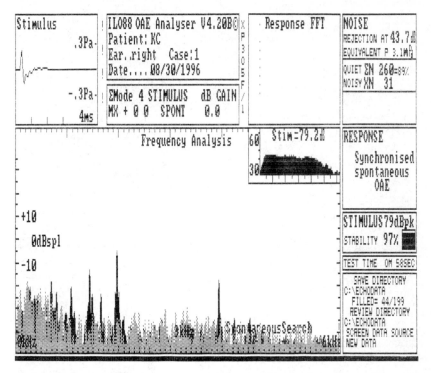

Fig 4-1. — Spontaneous otoacoustic emissions (SOAEs) recorded from an adult with normal hearing. The frequency range is marked on the X axis and the amplitude in dB SPL is marked on the Y axis. The gray areas represent the noise in the recording and the black spikes are the SOAE. The small box in the upper right corner shows the probe fit and stimulus level.

the basal, or high-frequency, portion of the cochlea responds first, because it is the first area activated by the signal, followed by the middle- and low-frequency areas as the traveling wave proceeds through the cochlea.

The difference between the two memory banks indicates the noise component. Noise can be either the patient's physiologic noise or ambient acoustic noise. Therefore, it is important that the patient and the environment be relatively quiet during testing. Although children tend to be noisier than adults, their TEOAEs tend to be larger. Therefore recordings can still usually be obtained.

The response is analyzed both graphically and numerically. When the response spectrum is plotted, the missing areas of the response correspond to areas of hearing loss and/or missing outer hair cells. Figure 4–2 displays a normal TEOAE response. The amplitude of the response is plotted in dB SPL on the ordinate and the spectrum of the response is plotted on the abscissa. The noise component is indicated

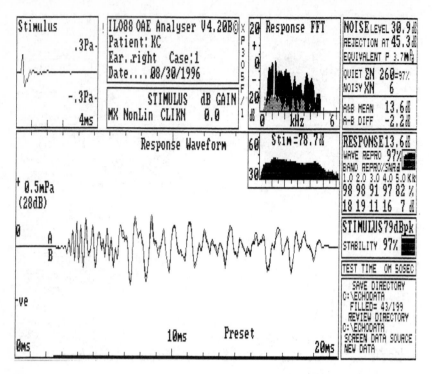

Fig 4-2. — Transient evoked otoacoustic emissions (TEOAEs) recorded from a normally hearing adult. The time domain recordings from memory banks A and B are overlapped in the bottom section. Note the excellent response replicability. The response spectrum is shown in the upper right-hand corner under "response FFT." The gray area represents the noise component and the black area represents the actual response. In the right column, from top to bottom is listed: the patient's noise level, the noise rejection level, then the number of accepted (quiet) responses, the number of rejected (noisy) responses, the A&B mean, which represents the amplitude of the response that correlates between memory banks A&B, the A-B difference which represents the amplitude of the noise component or the part of the recordings that did not correlate between memory banks A&B, the amplitude of the overall response is again listed, the reproducibility of the response, and then the reproducibility by frequency band and the amplitude of the response in each frequency band. In the upper left corner, the click stimulus is plotted in the time domain.

by the black area, and the response by the lighter area. The correlation representing the reliabilty of the response is charted for the overall response and for each octave band.

In general the TEOAE will be absent where ever peripheral sensorineural hearing loss exceeds approximately 30 dB HL. Therefore, if TEOAEs are present for all frequencies, cochlear function and peripheral hearing in that ear must be relatively normal. In some disorders (eg, ototoxicity and noise exposure), abnormalities in the TEOAEs may occur prior to changes in auditory threshold and can serve as an early warning sign of damage.

A conductive problem may preclude a TEOAE response even when the cochlea is functioning normally. TEOAEs will generally be absent in the presence of a flat tympanogram. Negative middle pressure may or may not preclude TEOAE recording. In some individuals with negative pressure up to −200 daPa, the TEOAE is present, but frequently with reduced amplitude; in others it is absent. Pressure equalization tubes do not appear to interfere markedly with TEOAE responses as long as hearing thresholds are normal and there are no air-bone gaps. However, TEOAE amplitude does negatively correlate with the size of air-bone gaps.

DPOAEs occur in response to two simultaneous tones of different frequencies presented to the ear. The lower frequency tone is called **F1** and the higher frequency tone is called **F2**. F2 is frequently, but not always, 1.21 times the frequency of F1. In response to F1 and F2 presentation, the ear generates other tones of different frequencies but with a clear frequency relationship to F1 and F2. These generated tones are called **"distortion products."** The largest distortion product is usually at the frequency that is two times the frequency of F1 minus the frequency of F2 or **"2F1 − F2."** Although 2F1 − F2 is of a much lower frequency than either F1 or F2, the presence/absence and/or amplitude of the 2F1 − F2 component correlates most closely with hearing thresholds at either the F2 frequency or approximately the midpoint between the F1 and F2 frequencies called the **"geometric mean."**

DPOAEs are usually graphed as either **"DP-grams"** as shown in Figure 4–3 for which the intensity of F1 and F2 is held constant and F1 and F2 are presented at different frequencies or as **"input-output functions,"** also called **"growth functions"** (Fig 4–4), in which the F1 and F2 frequencies are held constant, but are presented at different intensity levels.

Because tonal stimuli can be used for DPOAEs, the information obtained can be quite frequency specific and clinically useful. However, although DPOAE results do correlate with the frequency and degree of hearing loss, this relationship appears to be imperfect and more research is needed to determine specific criteria for predicting peripheral hearing loss on the basis of DPOAEs as well as the optimal recording parameters for those determinations.

SFOAEs are generated in response to an ongoing pure tone. Because the signal and the response overlap in time, the response is read as ripples in the recording. Therefore, the responses are difficult to interpret and are not currently used clinically.

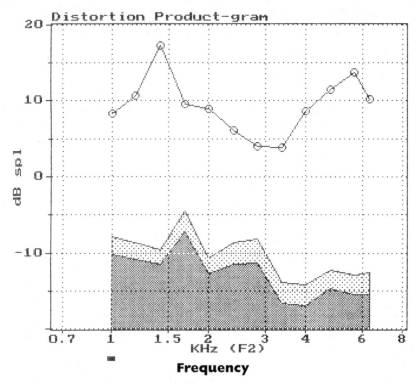

Fig 4-3. — Distortion Product Otoacoustic Emissions (DPOAEs) recorded from a normally hearing adult with FI and F2 held at 70 and 60 dB SPL, respectively. The frequency range (for F2) is marked on the X axis and the amplitude of the 2FI – F2 DPOAE is marked on the Y axis in dB SPL. The dark and cross hatched shaded areas represent one and two standard deviations of noise, respectively. The graph of DPOAEs plotted in this manner is sometimes called a "DP-Gram."

CLINICAL APPLICATIONS OF OAES

1. Site of lesion determination: Because OAEs are very specific to cochlear function (given a normal outer and middle ear), they can be very useful in differentiating between cochlear and retrocochlear lesion in sensorineural hearing loss. Additionally, OAEs can be useful in detecting cochlear damage before hearing threshold changes are observed (eg, ototoxic and noise-induced damage).

2. Hearing screening: As discussed in Chapter 3, OAEs and particularly TEOAEs have been recommended as a method of screening hearing in newborns. Some controversy exists regarding whether ABR or OAE screening is superior in terms of cost, personnel training, time,

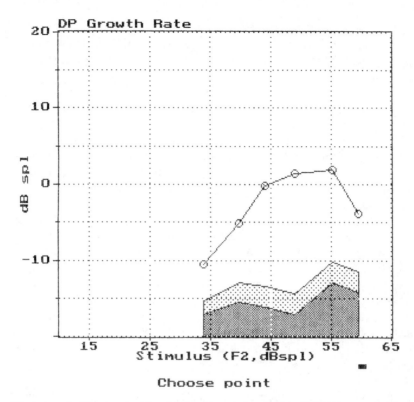

Fig 4-4. — An "input-output function" or "growth function" for DPOAEs recorded from a normally hearing adult with F2 held at 3000 Hz and F2 always 10 dB lower in intensity than F1. F2 intensity is marked on the X axis in dB SPL and the amplitude of 2F1 − F2 DPOAE is marked on the Y axis in dB SPL. The dark and cross hatched shaded areas represent one and two standard deviations of noise, respectively.

and accuracy. Essentially, both appear to be excellent methods of newborn hearing screening. ABR assesses the auditory pathway up through the level of the brainstem which is an advantage in that it tests a larger part of the auditory system and it is less affected by conductive disorders than OAEs. However, if the purpose of hearing screening is solely to detect peripheral (ie, cochlear hearing loss), then infants with neurologic disorder may be classified as "false positives" if the ABR abnormality is secondary to the neurologic lesion. OAEs are insensitive to neurologic abnormality but are more likely to be affected adversely by conductive problems, including debris in the ear canal, which can elevate the false positive rate. Additionally, some researchers assert that OAEs are faster and less expensive. Some reports recommend screening with one method and rescreening those that fail with the other method to avoid the false positives. A multitude of research studies are being carried out in this area to determine the optimal screening method and more recommendations are expected in the future.

3. Individual ear information in pediatric evaluations: As discussed in chapter 3, Pediatric Auditory Assessment, if there is an asymmetry of hearing between the two ears, behavioral sound-field hearing testing only provides information on the better ear. Therefore OAEs can be used to provide useful individual ear information quickly and objectively on cochlear function and OAEs are becoming a standard part of pediatric test batteries.

4. Assisting in "no response" ABR interpretation: When a threshold ABR yields no response even to high-level signals, the clinician cannot be certain if the ABR is absent because of peripheral hearing loss or because of neurologic dysfunction. If both OAEs and ABRs are absent (assuming normal outer and middle ear function), then peripheral hearing loss is most probably present and patient management can begin accordingly. If the OAEs are entirely normal and the ABRs are absent, the problem is neurologic and not attributable to peripheral hearing loss.

5. Ototoxic drug monitoring: OAEs may provide an early indication of ototoxic changes before actual threshold changes are observed. This information can allow the physician to consider other treatment options, possibly before hearing loss occurs. In children on ototoxic medications, OAEs can quickly provide individual ear information for monitoring whereas sound-field behavioral testing will only reflect hearing in the better ear.

6. Hearing aid candidacy determination: If OAEs are normal, any hearing loss observed is probably neurologic or inorganic (feigned or hysteric). Some clinicians recommend always testing OAEs before hearing aid fittings; other clinicians only test OAEs prior to hearing aid fittings in selected patient populations.

7. Inorganic hearing loss determination: Sometimes the clinician may suspect functional (feigned) or hysteric hearing loss. In these cases OAEs provide a quick, objective test of cochlear function. Frequently, after normal OAE results are obtained and explained to the patient (usually with the gentle suggestion that the patient must have misunderstood the instructions for the behavioral testing), reliable and accurate behavioral information can be obtained.

8. Hearing loss configuration confirmation: Particularly in cases of unusual or fluctuant hearing loss, OAEs can be used to determine if cochlear function matches the audiometric findings; the relationship is not always perfect but it can be helpful.

9. Efferent auditory system's function testing: Although not yet in common audiologic practice, contralateral suppression of TEOAEs shows promise for use in detecting extrinsic brainstem tumors (eg, lesions of the cerebello-pontine angle), particularly if they are compressing the brainstem, and appears to be very sensitive in detecting intrinsic brainstem lesions (eg, brainstem demyelination, brainstem infarct, olivo-ponto-cerebellar atrophy, syringomyelia, and arteriovenous malformation) (Prasher et al 1994.). Additionally, contralateral suppression has been shown to be reduced in Alzheimer disease, possibly secondary to the reduction of acetylcholine in that population (Campbell et al 1995). Research is continuing regarding the numerous possible clinical applications of contralateral OAE suppression.

Summary: OAEs are an extremely valuable tool for assessing cochlear function and in providing individual ear information. Because OAEs do not require a behavioral response from the patient, they can be evaluated even on a comatose patient. OAEs are particularly useful in site-of-lesion determination (including checking for feigned hearing loss), neonatal hearing screening, pediatric hearing testing, ototoxicity monitoring, and interpretation of "no response" ABRs.

Self-Assessment Questions

1. SOAEs are absent but TEOAEs have 70–85% replicability at all octave bands in a 21-year-old adult. What is your interpretation?

2. A neonate fails the otoacoustic emission screening but passes the ABR screening at a low intensity level. How do you interpret these findings?

3. A child with normal VRA results across all frequencies has normal TEOAEs in the right ear but absent TEOAEs in the left ear. What is your interpretation?

4. A 23-year-old musician has normal-hearing thresholds across the frequency range. However, the DP-gram shows a notch at 3–4 kHz. How do you interpret these findings?

5. A child has no ABR in either ear even for 90 dB nHL click stimuli, but the TEOAEs are normal. What is your interpretation?

Answers to Self-Assessment Questions

1. These results suggest bilaterally normal cochlear function. TEOAEs are generally absent when peripheral hearing loss exceeds approximately 30 dB HL. SOAEs may or may not be present in normals.

2. When the ABR screening results are normal and the otoacoustic emission screen is abnormal, the discrepancy is most probably the result of a conductive problem that has not elevated auditory threshold enough to cause an ABR abnormality but is preventing the otoacoustic emission from traveling from the cochlea back out to the ear canal to be detected by the probe microphone. Because the infant passed the ABR screen, there is very little chance of a permanent sensorineural hearing loss in the 2-4 kHz range.

3. The child probably has normal hearing in the right ear and either hearing loss and/or conductive disorder in the left ear. If tympanometry is normal in the left ear, the child probably has a sensorineural hearing loss in the left ear.

4. Although this patient currently has normal hearing, the notch in the DP-gram suggests hair cell damage and constitutes an early warning sign for further damage. The patient should be counseled regarding hearing protection.

5. This child probably has a neurologic disorder affecting the auditory pathway. The TOAEs suggest normal cochlear functioning, so hearing aids probably would not be recommended. However, some audiologists do recommend the trial of an auditory trainer for children with certain central auditory disorders (see Chapter 6).

References and Further Reading

1. Campbell KC, Hughes FL. A comparison of contralateral suppression of otoacoustic emissions in Alzheimer disease and matched control subjects. Abstracts of the Eighteenth Midwinter Research Meeting, *Association for Research in Otolaryngology*. 1995:70.
2. Decker N, ed. Otoacoustic emissions. *Sem Hearing*. 1992;13:1.
3. Prasher D, Ryan S, Luxon L. Contralateral suppression of transiently evoked otoacoustic emissions and neuro-otology. *Br J Audiol*. 1994;28:247-254.
4. Robinette M, Glattke T. *Otoacoustic Emissions: Clinical Applications*. New York: Thieme; 1997.

5

Electrophysiologic Measures: ECOG, ABR, and MLR

OVERVIEW: This chapter describes the various clinical auditory electrophysiologic measures including electrocochleography (ECOG), the auditory brainstem response (ABR), and a very brief description of the middle latency response (MLR). The late potentials are not discussed because they are not commonly used clinically at this time. This chapter focuses on the ABR because it is the response that is most widely used clinically. The basic science underpinnings are described only to the extent necessary to understand the clinical interpretation of the responses. The responses are described in the order they appear after the stimulus is presented to the ear. Because the acoustic stimuli used for evoked potentials are generally different than those used for behavioral audiometry, a brief discussion of the calibration references used is given.

CALIBRATION

The calibration for auditory evoked potential measures is very different than for pure-tone audiometry. The decibel is a relative measure and thus the reference must always be given. However, because very short duration (transient) stimuli must be used for evoked potentials, the decibel references used for pure-tone testing, which uses relatively long duration stimuli, are not usually appropriate for these measures. Each piece of equipment also must be individually calibrated, and clinicians should not simply rely on the "dial readings," which may not be accurate.

For auditory evoked potentials, the most commonly used references are nHL and peak equivalent SPL (pe SPL). For ABR click stimuli thresholds, the nHL value roughly predicts the HL audiometric values for the 2–4 kHz audiometric region. The pe SPL measure is used to attempt to equate a short duration signal to an equivalent longer duration pure-tone signal. Because these two references yield very different numerical values for the same test results, the physician must know the difference in reference values to interpret patient findings accurately. Usually, 0 dB nHL corresponds to 30 to 35 dB pe SPL (depending on lab norms). Therefore, a 30 dB nHL threshold may be equivalent to a 65 dB pe SPL threshold.

Each physician should also be aware that very short duration signals, as required for most auditory evoked potentials, do not have energy at just one frequency. Instead these signals have energy over a range of frequencies. Consequently, the results of auditory evoked potential testing are not as frequency specific as the results of pure-tone audiometry.

Some physicians will need more specific information regarding the signals and calibration used for auditory evoked potentials. Therefore, a brief calibration guide is provided at the end of this chapter.

ELECTROCOCHLEOGRAPHY (ECOG)

ECOG measures electrical activity from the cochlea and VIIIth nerve only. The response generally occurs in the first 5 ms after stimulus onset. An electrode is placed either in the ear canal, on the tympanic membrane, or through the tympanic membrane to touch the promontory over the cochlea and a reference electrode is generally placed on the vertex or contralateral earlobe or mastoid. A ground electrode is also used but its placement is less critical. Naturally, the closer the ipsilateral electrode is to the cochlea and/or VIIIth nerve, the larger the observed response will be and the better the signal-to-noise (S/N) ratio.

One important issue in electrocochleography is electrode selection. Transtympanic (TM) electrodes are a type of needle electrode placed through the tympanic membrane to rest on the promontory. These electrodes must be placed by a physician and require local anesthetic in adults and general anesthesia in children. Tympanic membrane electrodes have a foam or cotton tip and are placed directly on the tympanic membrane. They provide ECOG amplitudes about half as large as the transtympanic electrodes but do not require anesthesia. A variety of ear canal electrodes exists. The most commonly used ear canal electrode is the gold Tiptrode, which consists of a foam plug wrapped in gold foil with a hole in the center for signal delivery. The Tiptrode yields smaller ECOG recordings than the TM electrode but is very easy to place.

The **primary potentials recorded with ECOG** are the cochlear microphonic (CM), summating potential (SP), and compound action potential (AP or CAP).

Cochlear Microphonic (CM)

The CM is an AC microphonic potential that follows quite exactly the signal presented to the ear. It appears immediately when the signal stimulates the cochlea and continues throughout the stimulation. Therefore, if a sinusoidal stimulus is used, the CM will appear sinusoidal, and if a click stimulus is used, the CM will resemble the click stimulus. If you record the CM and play it back, you can actually reproduce the original signal. The primary problem in recording and interpreting the CM is that, if the signal and the CM overlap in time, it can be very difficult to distinguish the stimulus artifact radiating from the equipment from the CM. Because the CM is an AC potential, the CM and the stimulus artifact will be largely canceled out on the averaged recording when alternating polarity stimuli are used.

The CM is generated across the reticular lamina at the upper surface of the hair cells with the primary contribution, at least in normal ears, arising from the outer hair cells. The response follows the movement of the basilar membrane in response to an acoustic stimulus and is thus quite frequency specific. In research applications, the CM can be recorded from the scala vestibuli, the scala tympani, or the round window. However these recording sites are not practical clinically.

Although the clinician generally will not use the CM itself, it is important to be aware of the CM and recognize it as it may be present when recording other auditory evoked potentials.

Summating Potential (SP)

The SP is a DC potential, meaning that the response will be of a given polarity even when the stimulus polarity changes. It is observed as a unidirectional shift in the recording's baseline that lasts for the duration of the stimulus. Alternating polarity stimuli are frequently used to help cancel out the CM and stimulus artifact so that the SP can be measured more easily. The summating potential is generated by the hair cells, but the role the SP actually plays in hearing and specifically cochlear transduction of sound is not fully understood. SP amplitude is generally measured from the prestimulus baseline of the recording to the "kneepoint" of the SP, or to the point it joins the action potential (AP). In humans, SP polarity in a recording is frequently, but not always, the same as the AP.

Compound Action Potential (AP or CAP)

The AP is also referred to as the gross neural potential. Although individual neurons throughout the body and auditory system generate action potentials, in clinical auditory electrophysiology, the AP refers to the summed or averaged activity of action potentials of the VIIIth nerve in response to acoustic stimulation. The individual neurons' action potentials would be too small relative to the physiologic noise recorded with this electrode array to be observed in the recording. Therefore, the responses to approximately 1000 stimulations are averaged. Because noise is equally likely to be positive or negative at any point in time, noise "averages out" in the recordings. Although the firings of individual neurons will continue to occur throughout the acoustic stimulation, the AP will only be observed in response to the stimulus onset because that is when a high percentage of the neurons fire in synchrony. Only a synchronous response will create a clear waveform in the averaged response. Therefore, the AP is called an **"onset response"** and disorders that disrupt the neural synchrony of the VIIIth nerve may eliminate the AP, even when the patient can hear the stimulus.

The AP consists of two waveforms N_1 and N_2, which correspond to ABR Waves I and II. However, in ECOG in humans, frequently only N_1 is observed and only N_1 is used clinically.

Figure 5–1 shows an example of an electrocochleogram in a normal subject with the SP and AP marked.

Clinical Applications of ECOG

I. **Auditory Threshold Estimation:** The ECOG was commonly used to determine auditory threshold and still is used for that application

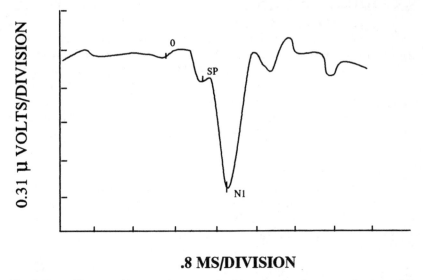

.8 MS/DIVISION

Fig 5-1. — Electrocochleogram in a normal subject showing the summating potential (SP) and action potential (AP)

in Japan and Europe. However, because a promontory electrode placement is generally used for the threshold determination, general anesthesia is also required, at least in children, which increases the risk and cost. With the advent of ABR with its noninvasive electrode placement, ECOG use for threshold determination fell into disuse. As described by Laureano et al 1995, ECOG with a TM electrode can be a useful adjunct in threshold determination in select applications, but is no longer commonly used for that purpose in the United States.

2. **Ménière's Disease and Perilymphatic Fistula:** In some clinics, ECOG is used as a part of the evaluation to detemine if a patient has either Ménière's disease or perilymphatic fistula. Essentially, the SP amplitude is compared to the AP amplitude and if the ratio is larger than normal, it is considered as indicative of Ménière's disease, although a perilymphatic fistula may also enlarge the SP/AP amplitude ratio. Definition of an "enlarged SP/AP amplitude ratio" varies from 0.3 to 0.5 to exceeding the 95% confidence interval in a normal population. Controversy exists regarding the sensitivity and specificity and thus the clinical utility of this measure, particularly in symptomatic patients with and without either Ménière's disease or perilymphatic fistula. Controversy also exists regarding the optimal electrode placement and recording parameters for this application. Research is continuing.

3. **ABR Wave I Identification:** Sometimes wave I of the ABR can be difficult to measure, particularly in a hearing-impaired patient. Yet, (as explained in the following section on ABR) wave I may be critical for the ABR analysis. The AP N_1 recorded in ECOG reflects the same activity as wave I of the ABR, but it is larger because the ECOG electrode placement is closer to the VIIIth nerve than the mastoid or earlobe placement commonly used in ABR. Using an ear canal electrode, which can be considered an ECOG electrode, for otoneurologic ABR applications is becoming common practice.

4. **Intraoperative Monitoring:** ECOG is being used for some applications in the operating room. Some clinicians place an electrode directly on the VIIIth nerve to monitor its function during acoustic neuroma excision. Others are investigating the SP/AP amplitude ratio during surgery for perilymphatic fistula.

5. **Cochlear implants:** Immediately after implantation, while the patient is still under anesthesia, electrically stimulated ECOG and/or ABR responses can be used to set an initial range for mapping cochlear implants, which can save time later, particularly in children. This application is still in development.

AUDITORY BRAINSTEM RESPONSE (ABR)

The ABR is also sometimes called the brainstem auditory evoked response (BAER) or the brainstem evoked response (BSER). The phrase "evoked response audiometry" (ERA) (which was usually used to refer to ABR, but sometimes to later potentials as well) has fallen into disuse because this test does not measure hearing directly but rather is a physiologic measure from which hearing status can be implied.

The ABR generally occurs in the first 10 ms after stimulus onset. Although the ABR can be recorded from a variety of electrode locations, most commonly an active electrode is placed at the vertex; the reference electrode is placed on the mastoid, earlobe, or in the ear canal; and a ground electrode is placed elsewhere. Usually recordings are obtained from both hemispheres simultaneously although typically only one ear at time is stimulated.

Like the AP in ECOG, the ABR is an onset response and requires synchronous neural discharges to produce clear waveforms. In humans, the ABR is characterized by seven waveforms, labeled sequentially by Roman numerals, although waves VI and VII have no known clinical utility.

Neural Generators

ABR measures the electrical activity along the auditory pathway from the VIIIth nerve to the lateral lemniscus and possibly the inferior colliculus. **Waves I** and **II** are generated by the distal and medial portions of the VIIIth nerve, respectively. **Wave III** is generated by the cochlear nucleus with perhaps some small contributions from nerve fibers entering the cochlear nucleus. **Wave IV** is generated from third-order neurons primarily from the superior olivary complex, but probably with additional contributions from the cochlear nucleus and the nucleus of the lateral lemniscus. Additional contributions to **waves III** and **IV** from other sources may also occur. **Waves V, VI,** and **VII** have complex neural generators, but the primary contributions for wave V appear to originate from the lateral lemniscus, while the primary generators for waves VI and VII appear to originate from the inferior colliculus.

ABR waveforms are labeled by convention with Roman numerals as shown in Figure 5–2.

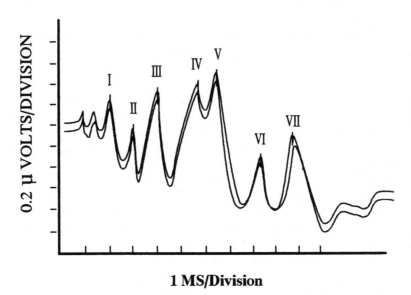

1 MS/Division

Fig 5–2. —The waveforms of the ABR are labeled by convention with Roman numerals. Although there are seven basic waveforms, only waves I, III, and V are generally analyzed in clinical work. The auditory brainstem response (ABR) from a normal adult subject with the primary waveforms labeled according to the Jewett scheme for peak labeling and with vertex positive up. (Please note that this is a representative ABR from a normally hearing individual and was obtained under optimal stimulus conditions. The appearance of even normal ABRs varies from individual to individual and learning to read and interpret them correctly usually requires considerable experience.)

ABR Measurements

Although the ABR comprises seven waveforms, usually only waves I, III, and V are analyzed for clinical work. Wave II, when clearly present, is sometimes analyzed, particularly for otoneurologic analysis, but wave II is more labile than waves I, III, and V and usually more difficult to measure.

Latency Measures

Absolute latencies are generally measured for waves I, III, and V particularly for all otoneurologic applications. **Absolute latency** is a measure of the time from stimulus onset to the peak of each wave. Waves I and III are measured at maximal peak, usually near the center of the waveform, but wave V is frequently measured at the last peak before the trough following wave V because waves IV and V frequently blend to some degree, which is called the **"IV–V complex."** Because of the travel time for the signal to reach and stimulate the VIIIth nerve, in response to a high-intensity click stimulus, wave I in a normal individual generally occurs at approximately 1.4 to 1.8 ms, with each of the subsequent waveforms following at approximately 1 ms intervals. Therefore, the **I–III interpeak interval** and the **III–V interpeak interval** are normally about 2 ms each and the I-V interpeak interval is normally about 4 ms long (Fig 5–3). When measurable, the I–II interpeak interval is approximately 1 ms. The **ILD V**, formerly called the IT_5, is the difference in absolute wave V latencies between the two ears. The normal ILD V is generally less than 0.3 ms. Sometimes an ILD V criterion value of 0.2 ms with correction factors for asymmetric hearing loss is employed.

Because normal values for the measurements depend on the stimulus and recording parameters, which can vary from clinic to clinic and for each piece of equipment, it is recommended that norms be obtained on 20 normally hearing individuals to establish means and standard deviations for each latency measure. Usually any value outside two standard deviations is considered to be abnormal. Because females tend to have slightly shorter latency values than males, some clinics obtain separate norms for females and males.

Waveform Presence or Absence

The presence or absence of waveforms I, III, and V is in itself important for interpretation. For example, if in response to a high intensity stimulus no waveforms are present after wave III bilaterally, a brainstem lesion may be present. If all waveforms are absent, the patient may

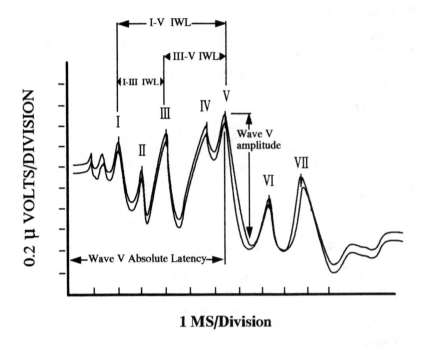

1 MS/Division

Fig 5-3. — Example of a normal ABR for an adult male. Shown is the Jewett scheme for peak labeling (vertex positive up) and the measurement of absolute and interpeak and interwave (IWL) latency and peak to trough amplitude.

have severe-to-profound hearing loss or a neurologic disorder. The presence or absence of wave V in response to stimuli of various intensities is generally used to determine ABR threshold and thus to imply hearing status. Waves I and III generally are not present in response to low-intensity stimuli, even in normals.

Absolute Amplitude Values

Absolute amplitude measures are so variable in humans that their clinical utility is limited. When absolute amplitude values are measured, they are usually taken from the peak of the waveform to the following trough.

Morphology

Although difficult to quantify, an experienced audiologist will be able to recognize when the ABR's form is not normal for a given patient and set of stimulus and recording conditions.

I/V Amplitude Ratios

Although absolute amplitude values are not generally useful, if wave I is substantially larger than wave V, the enlarged I/V amplitude ratio may be suggestive of retrocochlear lesion.

Rate Effects

Sometimes the stimulation rate is increased from approximately 10/s to a higher rate (eg, 50/s). If wave V shifts more than expected or disappears, it can be indicative of retrocochlear lesion (eg, multiple sclerosis).

Not all ABR measurements are used for all types of evaluations.

Clinical Applications of the ABR

1. **ABR threshold estimation:** ABR is commonly used to estimate the peripheral auditory sensitivity of a patient who cannot or will not cooperate for behavioral audiologic test procedures such as a child under 6 months of age, a developmentally delayed child, or an individual suspected of feigned hearing loss. This application is more fully discussed later in this chapter. (See ABR threshold estimation.)

2. **Otoneurologic assessment:** ABR can be used to determine if the auditory pathway from the VIIIth nerve to the lateral lemniscus is intact and firing synchronously. This application is more fully discussed later in this chapter (see ABR otoneurologic applications).

3. **Intraoperative monitoring:** ABR can provide intraoperative monitoring of the auditory pathway, particularly during procedures in which the status of the cochlea or VIIIth nerve could be affected either by interruption of the vascular supply, retraction, and/or direct manipulation (eg, acoustic neuroma excision). If the ABR suddenly shows latency prolongation or disappears, it is considered indicative of VIIIth nerve damage, which may be transient or permanent depending on the cause. Although facial nerve monitoring is almost invariably performed during these procedures, some clinics also routinely monitor the VIIIth nerve with ABR. Others feel that ABR monitoring does not significantly change the patient outcome and, therefore, do not routinely use it for this application.

4. **Monitoring the status of comatose patients and/or in brain death evaluations:** The presence of a normal ABR is a good prognostic sign for comatose patients. Some states require the use of ABR in

brain death evaluations. Naturally the absence of the ABR, suggesting brainstem damage, suggests a poor prognosis. In these cases, however, it is **absolutely essential** that the physician determine that the patient has essentially normal hearing at the time the ABR is performed. Hearing loss, either as a result of an acute injury or prior to the current medical condition, can also cause an absent ABR. The physician must also ensure that the patient's current medications could not affect the ABR. Acute alcohol intoxication or a history of chronic alcohol abuse can prolong ABR latencies and reduce ABR amplitude.

5. **Screening neonatal hearing:** ABR measures have been used for many years to screen hearing in neonates. Neonates usually are screened using a relatively low-intensity click stimulus (usually around 35 dB nHL). Frequently an automated screener (ALGO) that compares the infant's response to a template is used. If the ABR is present bilaterally, there is little likelihood of a handicapping hearing loss. If the ABR is absent in either ear, the infant is referred for follow-up testing. Studies are currently comparing the efficacy of ABR to otoacoustic emissions (OAEs) in screening infant hearing. At this time it appears that either method is effective. The ABR is well established and has good sensitivity and specificity for the detection of hearing loss, but the response can be absent in the case of neurologic disorder with normal hearing and usually takes longer than OAEs. OAEs are more time efficient, are not affected by neurologic disorder, but can be absent secondary to middle ear fluid and may be more easily affected by ambient noise in the test environment. Research in this area is continuing.

6. **Cochlear implants:** ABR threshold is determined, using electrical rather than auditory stimuli, immediately after cochlear implantation in children to obtain a starting point for mapping the electrodes. This application is still in development.

ABR Threshold Estimation

The ABR can be used to estimate auditory threshold in patients who cannot or will not cooperate for behavioral audiologic assessment. Usually ABR threshold evaluations are conducted in young children but they may also be used in legal cases, suspected feigned hearing loss, or in a comatose or developmentally delayed adult. The ABR does not measure actual hearing because true hearing involves the perception of sound and the ABR can be normal even in the absence of the auditory cortex.

ABR threshold is not interpreted in isolation. Several factors need to be considered including the patient's case history; the results of other audiologic tests including behavioral testing, otoacoustic emissions, and immittance audiometry; the patient's neurologic status; the patient's tympanic membrane and middle ear status; and the patient's age.

Click or tone burst stimuli can be employed. Pure-tone stimuli cannot be used because the ABR is an onset response requiring transient stimuli to elicit sufficient neural synchrony for an observable response. Thus, responses are not as frequency specific as in a pure-tone audiogram.

For click stimuli, normal ABR thresholds should be obtained at 30 dB nHL (approximately 60–65 dB pe SPL depending on clinic standards) or better. It is important for the physician to check the calibration reference being used for accurate interpretation of the threshold obtained. The ABR threshold in response to click stimuli usually corresponds to the 2–4 kHz region on the behavioral audiogram. Although the click stimulus has a very broad spectrum, it elicits an ABR response primarily from this relatively high-frequency region. This information is very useful because the 2–4 kHz region is critical for normal speech and language development. If hearing is normal in the 2–4 kHz range, hearing aids may not be fit, even if there is a substantial low-frequency hearing loss. An example of ABR threshold determination is provided in Figure 5–4. Note that, as signal intensity decreases, wave V latency increases, amplitude decreases, and waveform morphology blurs. Thus, the reponse can be more easily obscured by physiologic or acoustic noise. Therefore, replications are obtained, particularly near threshold, to ensure that a true response is present. Pseudoresponses resulting from noise, either physiologic or electric, will generally not replicate.

Frequency-specific stimuli can be used, but as described in the above section on calibration, the signals used for ABR cannot be as frequency specific as the pure tones used for behavioral audiometry. Tone burst stimuli of various frequencies can be used to provide an estimate of the configuration of the hearing loss. Sometimes noise, either noise with a notch around the center of the tone burst's frequency or various high-pass noise bands, can be used to improve the frequency specificity of the ABR. These procedures can ameliorate but not totally eliminate the problem. Because the clearest ABR waveforms are obtained in response to click or high-frequency tone burst stimuli, ABR estimates for low-frequency tone bursts (eg, 500 Hz) are not as accurate as for high-frequency threshold estimation. Because tone burst stimuli vary in duration and frequency content from clinic to clinic, each clinic must establish its own norms for the stimuli used.

The ABR cannot be tested on a vocalizing or active patient because the physiologic noise can obscure the response. Therefore, sedation,

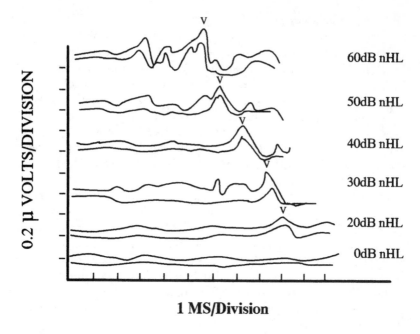

1 MS/Division

Fig 5–4. — An example of ABR responses at varying intensity levels for a normal subject. Using this method, with a replication at each intensity level, auditory threshold can be estimated by determining the lowest intensity level at which a replicable ABR response is still present.

commonly chloral hydrate, is frequently used for children from 6 months to 3–4 years old and for developmentally delayed individuals. Below 6 months of age, sedation is generally not needed because the infant can be tested during natural sleep periods.

Similarly ambient acoustic noise can obscure the response, and ABR threshold evaluations should be performed in a quiet, preferably sound-treated environment. When ABR threshold must be assessed outside of a sound-treated environment, noise reducing earphones or eartips can be used.

The child's age is a critical factor in interpreting the ABR. Usually an ABR will not be present in an infant under 28 weeks gestational age. When the ABR response first appears, its morphology is different than in the adult, and the waveform latencies are markedly prolonged. ABR latencies approximate adult values at approximately 1 year of chronological age (given a normal gestational period), but may not be fully at adult values until 2 years of age. Consequently, the child's age must always be considered when interpreting ABR latencies. ABR threshold can be screened at birth but diagnostic retesting and possible fitting of hearing aids is generally scheduled at 2 months of age (adjusted if the child was premature).

If the purpose of the ABR threshold evaluation is to determine permanent sensorineural hearing loss and the patient's candidacy for hearing aids, the child's tympanic membrane and middle ears should be healthy on the date of testing. Otherwise it will be difficult to determine how much of any hearing loss measured is secondary to a conductive and possibly transient problem. Bone-conducted signals can be used for ABR, and may be required for some cases (eg, Treacher-Collins syndrome), but determining air-bone gaps in ABR is not as accurate as in behavioral audiometry and sensorineural thresholds are best measured in the absence of conductive disorder.

For the child of 6 months or more developmental age, the ABR should be interpreted in conjunction with behavioral test results. For example, VRA results may suggest a mild hearing loss across the frequency range, but because VRA is tested in a sound field, VRA thresholds reflect only the hearing in the better ear. An important advantage of ABR (and also OAEs) is that objective individual ear information is obtained, which is critical for patient management including hearing aid fitting. However, ABR and behavioral information should be consistent with each other.

An absent ABR, even for high-level stimuli, can be indicative of either severe-to-profound hearing loss or neurologic disorder. In these cases, the clinician must test OAEs. If the ABR is absent and OAEs are normal, the patient probably has normal cochlear function and poor neural synchrony or other retrocochlear lesion. In this case hearing aid fittings may not be appropriate. However, if OAEs are also absent, the absent ABR may be secondary to hearing loss and hearing aids are indicated.

Otoneurologic Applications of ABR

ABR can be very useful in detecting retrocochlear disorders. As in the threshold evaluation, it is important that the patient be relaxed to reduce physiologic noise (eg, myogenic activity); however, in the cooperative adult, sedation is rarely required. For this application, a relatively high-intensity (around 85 dB nHL) click stimulus generally is used. The analysis includes computation of the I–III, III–V, and I–V intervals bilaterally as well as the ILD V. Because wave I is very useful for interpreting otoneurologic ABR evaluations, usually a gold Tiptrode, as described in the ECOG section of this chapter, is used to enhance wave I amplitude.

As discussed previously, it is essential that each clinic establish its own base of normal latency values from data obtained on 20 normal subjects. In many clinics, any measure outside 2 standard deviations is considered indicative of disorder. Usually the I–III and III–V interpeak intervals are approximately 2 ms and the I–V interval is approximately 4 ms. Prolongation (greater than 2 standard deviations) of the I–III interval suggests an VIIIth nerve lesion and a prolonged III-V interval suggests a lesion between the cochlear nucleus and the lateral lemniscus. However a cerebello-pontine angle tumor may also compress the brainstem causing signs consistent with a brainstem lesion not only on the side ipsilateral to the tumor but on the contralateral side as well. Prolongation of the I–III and/or III–V interpeak intervals will also prolong the I–V interval which is frequently used in the diagnosis of retrocochlear disorder. The ILD V is generally under 0.3 ms in normals as long as the peripheral hearing is symmetric between the two ears. However, patients frequently are referred for otoneurologic ABR because they have a unilateral or asymmetric hearing loss. Because conductive and/or sensorineural hearing loss can also prolong ABR absolute latencies, some clinicians use an ILD V criterion value of 0.2 ms with correction factors for the amount of hearing loss. Peripheral hearing loss will not, however, prolong ABR interpeak latencies and in fact in some cases may slightly shorten the I–V interpeak interval. Therefore, the interpeak intervals are more reliable in detecting retrocochlear lesion, than the ILD V, particularly in the presence of unilateral or asymmetric sensorineural hearing loss.

In the absence of wave I, the absolute wave V latency sometimes is compared to normal values to determine if it is prolonged. However, unless the hearing in that ear is normal, it can be difficult to determine if the wave V latency prolongation is secondary to retrocochlear lesion or peripheral hearing loss. In some cases, ABR waveforms may simply be absent secondary to retrocochlear lesion.

Because the neural generators of the ABR do not extend above the lateral lemniscus/inferior colliculus, thalamo-cortical lesions will not affect the ABR. The following are examples of expected ABR results in different types of retrocochlear lesions.

VIIITH NERVE AND CPA TUMORS. The most common of these tumors is the vestibular Schwannoma (often but inaccurately called acoustic neuroma). Usually these tumors will cause prolonged I–III and I–V intervals on the affected side and thus a prolonged ILD V. Sometimes the ABR is absent or only wave I is present. Sometimes wave I amplitude is substantially larger than wave V amplitude. If the lesion is compressing the brainstem, the contralateral side may show prolongation of the III–V and thus the I–V interval rendering the ILD V measure less useful because wave V is prolonged bilaterally. Brainstem compression can also result in contralateral absence of wave V. If the I–II interval can be measured on the ipsilateral side and is prolonged, the tumor is most probably intracanalicular. The physician must remember that these tumors can also interrupt cochlear blood supply, so signs of peripheral cochlear impairment may also be present and do not rule out the presence of a retrocochlear lesion.

NEUROFIBROMATOSIS 2 (NF 2). See VIIIth nerve and CPA tumors (above). However, in NF 2 patients, the incidence of acoustic neuromas is 95% and the tumors commonly are bilateral. Therefore, the I–V intervals may be prolonged bilaterally relative to normal values, but the ILD V may be less useful because of the bilateral abnormality.

BRAINSTEM LESIONS. These disorders (eg, pontine gliomas, brainstem neoplasms, and lesions compressing the brainstem) can yield ABR abnormalities usually involving bilaterally reduced, delayed, or absent wave Vs with or without concomitant abnormalities of wave III.

LEUKODYSTROPHIES Leukodystrophies can cause a variety of ABR abnormalities, including delayed waveforms, prolonged I–V interpeak latencies, and absence of waveforms, particularly waves III through V with I and II sometimes remaining.

MULTIPLE SCLEROSIS (MS). The ABR is less sensitive than visual or somatosensory evoked potentials in detecting MS because the plaques are more likely to affect those pathways. However, several abnormalities of the ABR can occur, as can hearing loss secondary to MS, and ABR can thus serve as one of the corroborating factors for diagnosing the disease. Depending on where the plaques occur along the auditory pathway, abnormalities may be unilateral or bilateral. When the ABR is abnormal, most frequently interpeak latencies will be markedly affected or later waveforms may simply be absent. Increasing stimulation rate may cause a marked wave V latency shift or disappearance of waveforms. Patients with optic neuritis, who subsequently may develop MS, may or may not have similar ABR abnormalities.

VASCULAR DISORDERS. Vascular disorders frequently mimic the findings for vestibular Schwannomas. However, depending on the location and type of vascular disorder, a number of different ABR abnormalities may be produced.

Many other disorders can cause ABR abnormalities. The reader is referred to the excellent texts listed at the end of this chapter for further reading.

MIDDLE LATENCY RESPONSES (MLRS)

The MLR is an onset response with the primary waveforms occurring 15–60 ms after the stimulus. The MLR has broader waveforms and larger amplitude than the ABR. The MLR is generated in the thalamo-cortical region of the auditory pathway. The primary waveforms are Na, Pa, and Nb, Pb (Fig 5–5). Although the MLR has been known for several decades, its clinical applications are still under investigation. The MLR can be used in adults to estimate auditory threshold, sometimes simultaneously with the ABR. However, whether the MLR is reliable in children is controversial and children comprise the primary patient population for threshold estimation. Another clinical limitation is that, unlike the ABR, the MLR is highly dependent on sleep state and is best recorded in a relaxed but awake patient.

Otoneurologic applications exist but are not as well defined as for the ABR. Lesions of the thalamo-cortical areas can affect MLRs, but insufficient literature exists currently for exact categorization of results. Also, lower level lesions (eg, vestibular Schwannoma) can cause MLR abnormalities, as can peripheral hearing impairment.

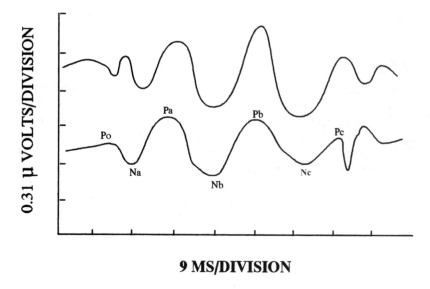

9 MS/DIVISION

Fig 5-5. — The middle latency response (MLR) from a normal adult showing designation of the primary waveforms.

A BRIEF GUIDE TO CALIBRATION REFERENCES FOR EVOKED POTENTIALS

Intensity References for Auditory Evoked Potentials

The decibel is a relative measure, thus the reference must always be given. Physicians are frequently familiar with SPL and HL but are less familiar with calibration references for evoked potentials. Physicians must be familiar with these references to interpret test results properly and evoked potential equipment should be calibrated regularly. Over time, the constant pounding of transient signals on transducers can damage earphones.

Signals selected for evoked potentials generally need to be of a short duration with a fast rise/fall time to elicit the onset response. However, there is a **reciprocal relationship** between the duration of the signal and the spectral spread of energy. The shorter the duration, the wider the spectral spread of energy in the frequency domain. Therefore, the shorter the duration of the signal, the more likely it is to elicit clear waveforms because it will cause neurons to fire synchronously, but at the cost of frequency specificity. Therefore there is always a tradeoff between the short signal duration needed to elicit the onset response and the desire for a frequency-specific signal.

dB nHL

0 dB nHL corresponds to the behavioral threshold of a group of 10–20 normally hearing listeners for the exact stimulus being employed for evoked potentials. 0 dB nHL for clicks generally corresponds to approximately 30–35 dB peSPL, but varies slightly from lab to lab because of differences in equipment, stimuli, and slight differences between normally hearing listeners. The nHL reference is commonly used only for click stimuli. The nHL reference is not very useful for tone burst stimuli because the behavioral threshold for tone bursts is highly dependent on the tone burst duration (eg, the longer the duration of the tone burst, the lower the behavioral threshold), whereas the threshold of auditory evoked potentials, such as ECOG and ABR, does not improve as signal duration is increased.

dB peSPL

The peSPL (peak equivalent sound pressure level) reference is generally used for click stimuli. For this measure, the acoustic output from the transducer is fed into a sound level meter and the output from the sound level meter is then fed into an oscilloscope. The amplitude of the click stimulus is measured in volts from prestimulus baseline to the peak of the first (largest) excursion of the click stimulus. That amplitude is then matched to the same amplitude measure of a pure-tone stimulus of known SPL. Therefore, a 100 dB peSPL signal has equivalent amplitude, as measured using this method, to a 100 dB SPL pure-tone signal. The frequency of the pure-tone reference is frequently either 1000 Hz or a frequency approximating the peak resonant frequency of the transducer being employed.

dB SPL

The SPL reference is generally used for tone-burst signals. However, most sound level meters cannot adequately measure the SPL of tone bursts because the duration is too short. Therefore, for calibration purposes, either the duration of the tone burst is lengthened so that the SPL can be measured with the sound level meter or the tone burst's plateau amplitude is measured, usually from maximally negative to maximally positive peak, and then matched to that of a pure-tone signal.

HL and **SL** values are generally not optimal measures for calibrating transient signals for clinical use.

Frequency References for Auditory Evoked Potentials

Stimulus frequency must be measured with a spectrum analyzer. Frequency counters are inadequate because of the spectral spread of energy of the transient signal.

Tone bursts are described by their center frequency. Their plateau, rise/fall time, and transducer will then dictate the spectral spread of energy, but the spectrum must be checked on the spectrum analyzer to ensure that the frequency content is as desired. The **gating function**, or the way the signal is turned on and off, is also important in the spectral spread of energy. A linear gating function produces essentially a straight line during the rise/fall times. Turning the signal on with a curved gating function (eg, a cosine squared or Blackman gating function) helps reduce the spread of spectral energy.

For clicks, the duration of the click and transducer will dictate its spectrum. For example, the main lobe of a 100 µs click will extend to a null point of 10 kHz, but the transducer will act as an output filter further shaping the spectrum.

Summary: Auditory electrophysiologic measures can provide excellent information on auditory site-of-lesion, otoneurologic status, and auditory screening and threshold determination, including individual ear information. Depending on the potential measured, auditory electrophysiologic measures can reflect activity from the cochlea up to and including the auditory cortex. Because most electrophysiologic measures do not require a behavioral response from the patient, information can be obtained even on a comatose patient.

Self-Assessment Questions

1. A 2-month-old infant has ABR click thresholds of 20 dB nHL bilaterally. What is your interpretation?

2. An adult patient has normal pure-tone air-conduction audiometric thresholds. ABR waves I and III are bilaterally normal, but wave V is absent bilaterally. What is your interpretation?

3. A 6-month-old child has no ABR in either ear at 100 dB nHL. What is your interpretation?

4. An adult patient with a unilateral mild sensorineural hearing loss in the right ear has a markedly prolonged I–V interval on the that side. On the left side the I–III interval is normal, but the III–V interval is markedly prolonged. What is your diagnosis?

5. A 2-month-old infant has ABR click thresholds at 55 dB peSPL bilaterally. What is your interpretation?

Answers to Self-Assessment Questions

1. These thresholds suggest essentially normal hearing bilaterally for the 2000 Hz to 4000 Hz frequency range.

2. These results would be suggestive of a brainstem lesion. Results like these could be observed with a space occupying lesion (eg, pontine glioma) or other disorders affecting the brainstem (eg, vascular disorder, or possibly MS.)

3. This child could have profound hearing loss bilaterally or could have neural dysynchrony. Otoacoustic emission testing would be essential for differential diagnosis.

4. These findings would be suggestive of a vestibular Schwannoma (or a similar lesion) on the right side that is compressing the brainstem and thus affecting the findings for the left side.

5. These results are the same as for question #1. Because 55 dB peSPL is equal to 20 to 25 dB nHL (depending on lab norms), these results are bilaterally normal.

References and Further Reading

1. Hall JW. *Handbook of Auditory Evoked Responses.* Boston: Allyn and Bacon; 1992.
2. Jacobson, JT, ed. *The Auditory Brainstem Response.* San Diego Calif: College-Hill Press; 1985.
3. Jacobson JT, ed. *Principles and Applications in Auditory Evoked Potentials.* Boston: Allyn and Bacon; 1994.
4. Laureano AN, McGrady M, Campbell K. Comparison of tympanic membrane electrocochleography and the auditory brainstem response in threshold determination. *Am J Otolaryngol.* 1995;16(2):209-215

6

Hearing Aids

OVERVIEW: This chapter describes the selection of hearing aid candidates, the various styles and types of hearing aids available, their components, their output characteristics, and fitting methods. Auditory trainers are briefly described. Cochlear implants and tactile aids are discussed in Chapter 7.

SELECTION OF HEARING AID CANDIDATES

The audiologist considers several factors in determining hearing aid candidacy. One of the factors is the patient's hearing loss, but intimately related to that is the patient's perception of that hearing loss. Even patients with a very mild hearing loss or a hearing loss restricted to the high frequencies can benefit from amplification. However, if no hearing loss is present in the 2 to 3 kHz range, most patients will not accept hearing aids even if they have hearing loss above or below that frequency range. Because most hearing losses occur gradually, many patients will not be aware of how much they are missing, even though their family members may complain. However, most patients will not try hearing aids unless they personally believe they are having trouble. Others, once they have tried hearing aids, report that they thought they were doing well before but now "it's easy." In general, even patients with a mild hearing loss should be encouraged to try amplification. Patients may adjust to hearing aids more easily if they are fitted soon after the onset of the hearing loss while they still retain quick recognition of all the speech sounds and while they are still used to background noise. However, patient motivation and realistic expectations are critical to success. Trying to force a patient to accept hearing aids, however well intentioned, is rarely successful. Patients who want hearing aids only for difficult situations (eg, the occasional party) will probably never adjust to the use of amplification. Although many patients readily accept wearing glasses, many still feel that there is a stigma attached to wearing hearing aids. These concerns should be discussed in advance of the fitting.

In most cases, hearing aid candidates have sensorineural hearing losses because most conductive hearing losses can be corrected medically and/or surgically. Although hearing aids are generally beneficial, they will not return hearing to normal because sensorineural hearing losses usually distort any signal presented to the ear and are frequently accompanied by recruitment. Conductive hearing losses do not generally distort sound and are not accompanied by recruitment. Therefore patients with conductive hearing losses usually do very well with amplification. Conductive hearing losses are typically fitted with hearing aids only when the condition is chronic and when medical/surgical treatment is ineffective. Amplification may be helpful for children having chronic middle ear problems.

Patients with unilateral hearing loss may or may not want a hearing aid. If the patient is frequently in group listening situations or other challenging communication environments, he or she may definitely want amplification. Other patients in less demanding communicative environments may not feel handicapped by a unilateral loss and may not desire amplification.

Most patients with bilateral hearing loss will obtain optimal benefit, particularly for difficult listening environments, from binaural hearing aid fittings. Binaural hearing aid fittings can provide **binaural summation**, which is hearing threshold improvement that occurs when listening with two ears as opposed to one ear. Binaural hearing aids can also provide **binaural squelch**, which is the ability to "tune out" unwanted noise. Additionally, the patient with two hearing aids will not be forced to favor the aided ear in most listening situations. However, finances and communicative needs also must be considered.

Children with bilateral hearing loss are almost always fitted with binaural hearing aids unless the hearing in one ear is so much poorer than in the other ear that amplifying the poorer ear could degrade overall performance. Binaural amplification for children is especially important to optimize the their acquisition of speech and language and to stimulate the central auditory pathways so that they will develop normally. Early identification of hearing loss is critical. Whenever possible, hearing aids are fitted as young as 2 months of age.

HEARING AID STYLES

Over the years, microcircuitry has developed to the point that a wide variety of hearing losses can be fitted with a variety of hearing aid styles. Naturally, there is a correlation between the amount of available circuitry and the size of hearing aid casing, but this limitation is less of a factor than in earlier decades. Nonetheless, there are some basic considerations in selecting hearing aid style:

1. Usually, the larger the hearing aid the greater the number of circuitry options available, including the amount of gain (amplification), noise suppression circuitry, methods of controlling the maximum power output (MPO), and telecoils for telephone coupling.
2. Traditionally, the farther the microphone is from the hearing aid's output into the ear canal, the less the likely it is to generate feedback. **Feedback** is the whistling sound that hearing aids produce when the hearing aids' output is fed back into the input and reamplified. Feedback can usually, but not always, be prevented by a snug fit of the hearing aids or earmolds into the ear canals. Regardless of fit, most hearing aids will feed back when covered, as with a scarf or a pillow. Feedback will also occur if a hearing aid is left on when it is out of the ear. Leaving the hearing aid on also increases battery drain, and feedback has caused many a dog to destroy hearing aids.
3. For analog hearing aids, the larger the hearing aids, the fewer the number of repair problems. Programmable and digital hearing aids

are predicted to have a longer life span and fewer repairs than analog hearing aids, irrespective of size, but they are still too new on the market to have yielded adequate long-term data.

4. Often, the smaller the hearing aids, the more difficult they are to manipulate. Patients with visual or manual dexterity problems may have difficulty inserting or removing some miniature hearing aids, adjusting the volume controls or telecoils, or changing the batteries. Because most hearing aid batteries need to be changed every 7 to 10 days, it is important for patients or their caregivers to be able to change the batteries themselves.

5. Technology and options should always be matched to the patient's ability to understand and consistently use the options.

The **basic styles of hearing aids** (Fig 6–1) and **some fitting considerations** follow.

Completely-in-the-Canal Aids (CICs)

These are extremely small hearing aids that fit deeply into the ear canal. They can only be seen when looking directly into the ear canal. CICs can only be fitted to mild-to-moderate hearing losses, but some noise control circuitry can be included. Advantages include the cosmetic appeal, probable reduction of the occlusion effect, virtual elimination of wind noise (the sound of wind blowing across the microphone), feedback reduction, greater high-frequency gain, enhanced comfort and freedom (especially for active patients), improved telephone use, and the ability to test each aid under an earphone in hear-

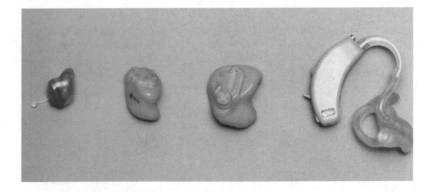

Fig 6–1 — A photograph showing four of the most common hearing aid styles. From left to right, a completely-in-the-canal aid hearing aid (CIC), a canal hearing aid, an in-the-ear hearing aid, and a behind-the-ear hearing aid (BTE)

ing testing. However, some patients dislike the sensation of the deep placement and others have difficulty manipulating the devices, particularly patients with manual dexterity problems because CICs must be removed by pulling on a small filament extending from the hearing aid. However, some patients with manual dexterity or visual problems actually find CICs easier to use than other hearing aid styles. Batteries may be difficult to change. CICs usually have no volume control although some automatic circuitry can help compensate for the absence of a volume control. Many patients actually prefer not having to adjust the volume. Telecoils cannot be fitted into CICs but a telephone usually can be used directly with the CIC hearing aids.

Canal Hearing Aids

Canal aids are larger than CICs. They basically fill the entire ear canal, but do not extend as deeply in the canal as CICs, nor do they fill the concha portion of the external ear. Canal hearing aids, because they are larger, have more circuitry options than CICs but still are generally only appropriate for mild-to-moderate hearing losses. Options for noise suppression circuitry and maximum power output controls (see following section on controls) may be somewhat limited. Canal aids generally have volume controls, but not telecoils. Individuals with small or collapsing canals may not be able to wear either CIC or canal hearing aids. Vents to provide ventilation, pressure reduction, or alteration of the acoustic signal can sometimes, but not always, be included in canal hearing aids. Because the microphone is so close to the hearing aid's output, the likelihood of feedback is higher than with larger hearing aids.

In-the-Ear Hearing Aids (ITEs)

In-the-ear hearing aids are extremely popular. ITEs may fill the concha portion of the outer ear (full shell) or only the bottom half (half shell). These aids have their circuitry housed in the concha portion of the hearing aid although they also have a canal portion for signal delivery. Most hearing losses can be fitted with ITE hearing aids, and several circuitry and venting options are available for them.

Behind-the-Ear Hearing Aids (BTEs)

BTEs hang behind the pinnae and are attached to **earmolds**, custom-made pieces that fit into the conchae and ear canals for signal delivery. With improvements in the smaller hearing aids, BTEs are no longer as popular as they were in the past, but they do have several advantages. In general, BTEs have fewer repair problems and less chance of feedback. Patients who perspire a great deal (eg, outdoor workers, gardeners, or athletes) may have problems with moisture build-up and/or corrosion with smaller hearing aids. With BTEs, most of the moisture will accumulate in the earmold, which can be removed, cleaned, and dried. Patients with chronic otitis externa or other skin problems affecting the ear canal or pinnae may be able to wear a BTE with an open (nonoccluding) earmold or other earmold fitting when ITEs, ITCs, or CICs are inappropriate. Some patients still prefer BTEs cosmetically, because if hair is styled over the BTEs, the earmolds are frequently less visible than ITEs.

Children, younger than 9 to 12 years of age, are almost always fitted with BTEs with soft earmolds. BTEs are very sturdy and usually need fewer repairs, which is important because children are very hard on hearing aids. With BTE hearing aids, the child can frequently use a loaner hearing aid attached to his or her earmold during the repair period, but this is not possible with other styles unless earmolds have been made in case of such situations. Also, as children grow, their ear canals and pinnae also grow. With BTE hearing aids, only the earmolds need to be changed (about every 6 months). With an ITE hearing aid, the entire hearing aid has to be sent in for recasing, which is much more expensive, and the child loses the use of the hearing aid during that time. Some manufacturers are sensitive to these issues and are willing to remake other styles of hearing aids without charge, but this benefit usually extends only during the warranty period.

The most important factor in fitting children with BTEs is safety. ITEs can have a soft canal portion but the circuitry must be housed in a hard plastic shell. If a child is hit in the ear while wearing an ITE, it can shatter into the pinna and/or ear canal. This problem can be avoided with BTE hearing aids with a soft earmold. Additionally, young children's ears are generally too small to allow for adequate circuitry in canal or ITE hearing aids.

Body Style Hearing Aids (Body Aids)

Body aids, which are approximately the size of a cigarette case, are still available but rarely used. They are very durable and provide maximal separation of the microphone and receiver and thus may be useful for children with very poor head control and feedback problems, particularly with profound hearing loss. They also can be used with children whose pinnae are inadequate to support BTE hearing aids or for children with no external ear canal (eg, infants with Treacher-Collins syndrome). In the latter case, a body aid can be attached to a bone-conduction delivery system to facilitate speech and language development. One of the problems with body aids is microphone placement. Because the microphone is not at ear level, the signal can be attenuated by body baffle, in which the mass of the patient's body reduces the input to the hearing aid. Additionally, input to the microphone can be noisy or reduced by interference of the patient's clothing. Ear-level microphone placement is preferable because most speech signals are directed to the patient's face.

Eyeglass Hearing Aids

These hearing aids are no longer generally available but physicians may occasionally still see one in use. Basically, the hearing aid circuitry was housed in the temple portions of eyeglasses. Consequently, the temple portions were large and generally unattractive. Attempting to shape the temples for the eyeglass fitting frequently damaged the circuitry. Although this style was popular for cosmetic reasons in the early 1970s, it was soon realized that it had several disadvantages. The most important disadvantage was that the hearing aids and eyeglasses were connected, and when one device broke, both were lost during the repair period.

"Bubble" Hearing Devices

These hearing aids have no electrical components, but rather are plastic shells custom fit into the pinna and ear canal and then hollowed out to provide some mid- to high-frequency resonance (between 1000 Hz to 2000 Hz). Above 2000 Hz, these devices attenuate the signal. Understandably, they have not become popular but physicians may hear of them. Because they do not require batteries and have no working parts, they could be useful in geographic locations with very limited technological support. Generally, they provide little more gain than cupping a hand behind the ear.

Contralateral Routing of Signal (CROS) Hearing Aids

CROS hearing aids look like bilateral hearing aid fittings but have only one microphone placed on one side with the signal then routed to the other side. The side without a microphone usually has a nonoccluding earmold so that the patient can still hear naturally on that side. CROS hearing aids are usually fitted when a patient has a deaf ear on one side and fairly normal hearing on the other. The open earmold does provide some slight high-frequency resonance. This resonance may be helpful if the patient has a slight high-frequency hearing loss in the better ear. The primary purpose of fitting CROS hearing aids is to eliminate the **head shadow effect.** The head shadow effect occurs when the high-frequency portion of the signal presented on the side of the poorer ear is attenuated by the mass of the patient's head before it arrives at the far ear.

Sometimes CROS hearing aids are used when the poorer ear is not completely deaf, but presents a signal so distorted that it degrades overall speech perception. In cases of severe recruitment and poor word recognition (eg, Ménière's disease), the patient may prefer a CROS to an ipsilateral hearing aid fitting. The CROS fitting allows the patient to hear signals presented on both sides without constantly having to position the better ear near the speaker. Although the CROS hearing aid does not provide true localization of sound, many patients can tell which side the sound is on because of the difference in sound quality from the sound routed through the microphone and the sound received directly from the environment.

Typically, patients prefer CROS hearing aids in which the microphone on the poorer ear transmits the signal via radio frequency (RF) transmission to a receiver on the other ear. Hard wires can be substituted for RF technology if needed (eg, the patient works in a high-RF environment); however, many patients defer the use of amplification if this is their only option.

Bilateral Routing of Signal (BICROS)

The BICROS is like a CROS but has a microphone that provides amplification on the better side in addition to a microphone on the poorer ear. This fitting is used when the patient has one aidable and one unaidable ear.

Ipsilateral Routing of Signal (IROS)

The IROS is not a CROS hearing aid but rather an ipsilateral hearing aid fitted to an ear with a nonoccluding earmold or simply tubing bent into the ear canal. The nonoccluding (open) earmold basically provides only high-frequency amplification. Therefore, this type of fitting is sometimes used for steeply sloping high-frequency hearing losses. Because the open earmold allows the amplified signal to be picked up by the microphone and reamplified, feedback can be problematic for all but mild hearing losses. With advances in hearing aid circuitry, hearing aid outputs can be shaped more precisely to hearing losses than in the past, and audiologists are less dependent on modifying the hearing aid output by earmold modifications. Therefore, IROS fittings have become less common for frequency shaping. The open earmold can be helpful for patients who need a well-ventilated ear canal and have a high-frequency, sloping hearing loss.

CRISCROS

Theoretically, CRISCROS hearing aids deliver signals received on the right side to the left ear and vice versa. The purpose of this fitting is supposedly to reduce feedback. However, better methods currently exist to reduce feedback problems, thus the arrangement is rarely used today.

Auditory Trainers

Auditory trainers are personal or group amplification systems used frequently in classroom settings to enhance the signal-to-noise ratio (S/N) for persons having hearing losses by effectively reducing the distance between the talker's and listener's ears. Historically, auditory trainers employed hard wire systems in which the child was linked to the teacher (ie, the teacher's microphone was wired to the child's receiver). Although this system improves S/N, it limits mobility. Loop systems are also used with auditory trainers, wherein the room is wired in a loop arrangement, the speaker talks with a microphone, and the listener can adjust personal hearing aids having telecoils to the "T" position (or use special receivers). Although loop systems also enhance the S/N and provide a good quality signal, they too limit mobility and signals may leak or spill over into adjacent classrooms. Modern auditory trainers operate via FM transmission systems, linking a microphone (transmitter) placed next to the speaker (eg, the child's teacher) to the child's own receiving system. This method reduces or eliminates much of the ambient noise that could interfere with the speaker's voice with standard hearing aids and allows the teacher to be heard without shouting across the room, while enhancing the S/N and reducing mobility problems. Auditory trainers may be housed in body-style or ear-level casings. Some auditory trainers attach to the child's hearing aids. Most auditory trainers can be set to receive only FM, only the microphone input, or both simultaneously. Auditory trainers are most commonly used with profoundly hearing-impaired children, but those with less severe hearing losses may benefit from the improved S/Ns that auditory trainers provide. Newer applications include using auditory trainers with only minimal amplification for children with normal-hearing sensitivity but with central auditory processing disorders. Because these children may have difficulty understanding in background noise, the direct FM signal may be helpful to them.

HEARING AID COMPONENTS

Hearing aids consist of a **microphone** that transduces incoming acoustic signals to electric energy, an **amplification stage,** and an output transducer (called a **receiver**) that converts the electrical signal back into an acoustic signal. Over the years, not only have hearing aids become miniaturized but hearing aid circuitry has improved considerably. The sensitivity and fidelity of microphones and receivers have markedly improved. Some hearing aids use **directional microphones** and/or multimicrophone arrangements that are more sensitive to signals arriving in front of the microphone than to signals arriving from behind the microphone. **Telecoils (telephone induction pickups)** that detect the magnetic field from telephones are available in a greater variety of hearing aids now. Previously, many hearing aid users did not like telecoils because of their poor fidelity and insensitivity to many telephone outputs. However, new telecoils approximate the characteristics of hearing aid microphones, and special adapters have been developed to amplify telephone signals. The amplification stage has also been markedly improved over the years, especially with nonlinear circuitry. Current hearing aids provide far less distortion, improved fidelity, enhanced battery life, and improved cosmetic appeal over hearing aids of the past. In addition, the amount of amplification for each frequency can be selected and more precisely fitted to the hearing loss, both because of improved hearing aid technology and improved fitting methods.

Traditionally, most hearing aids included **linear analog circuitry,** but the introduction of **nonlinear, programmable,** and **digital technology** currently provides many new options. Analog hearing aids have solid state circuitry that can be adjusted only by physical modification of the circuit setting by the manufacturer, or by resetting a potentiometer with a screwdriver, or turning the volume control, but usually only within a limited preset range. Programmable hearing aids allow the hearing aids to be set via computer control, providing a much wider range of settings for a given hearing aid. If the patient's hearing changes, programmable hearing aids can often be reset easily in the audiologist's office rather than having to be sent back to the manufacturer for modification or requiring the purchase of new hearing aids. Patients may also be able to carry a remote control that allows them to reset the hearing aids according to the listening environment. Presently, only a few manufacturers offer truly digital hearing aids that employ digital signal processing (DSP), which offers almost unlimited options and enhanced clarity and comfort for patients. Digital hearing aids undoubtedly will become more popular in the future. Some programmable and digital hearing aids constantly sample the input signal to adjust the hearing aids' output automatically to the patient's most comfortable listening level. Additionally, programmable and digital hearing aids can provide many other options for sophisticated signal processing, which are not available in simple analog hearing aids. However, some patients may not be able to afford the extra cost of programmable and digital hearing aids or may not need the extra technology.

DESCRIPTORS OF HEARING AID PERFORMANCE

Hearing aid performance can be measured in many ways. The basics of these measurements are described in the following section to enhance physicians' ability to communicate better with audiologists regarding patients' fitting requirements. These measurements can be applied to both analog and programmable hearing aids.

Gain

Gain describes the amount of amplification provided by the hearing aid. Gain is the difference between the hearing aid's input and output sound pressure level (SPL). For example, if the hearing aid's input is a 20 dB SPL signal at 1000 Hz and the hearing aid's output is 60 dB SPL at 1000 Hz, the hearing aid's gain at 1000 Hz is 40 dB SPL. However, gain may be measured in several ways. Some measures of gain are obtained in a special hearing aid test chamber called an automatic test device, more commonly referred to as a **hearing aid analyzer** or **test box**. For most of these measures, the hearing aid is attached to a special coupler (frequently a 2 cc coupler that approximates human ear canal volume, but special couplers are available), a calibrated signal that sweeps across frequencies at 50 or 60 dB SPL is presented, and the hearing aid's output in response to the input signal is read out by a calibrated microphone. Although gain can be computed at each frequency from these measures, often the "HFA gain" or "high frequency average gain" is reported which is the averaged amount of gain at 1000, 1600, and 2500 Hz. Although the HFA gain is usually tested with the volume control of the hearing aid full on, the hearing aid's **frequency response** is generally tested in a similar manner but with the volume control at a reduced setting. The hearing aid's frequency response is the amount of gain it provides at the various frequencies, or the shape of its output frequency spectrum. Other measures (eg, distortion, battery drain, equivalent input noise, telecoil measures etc.) are frequently obtained along with the gain measures in the hearing aid test box, but most physicians will not desire in-depth detail regarding these tests.

Functional gain is the measure of patients' sound-field thresholds with and without the hearing aids in place. As described below, real-ear measurement systems have largely replaced functional gain measures, but they are still useful for some patients. **In situ hearing aid gain** measurements reflect the amount of hearing aid gain at the eardrum. These measurements may be made on the patient using a small probe microphone in the patient's ear canal (**real-ear measures**) or may be **"simulated in situ"** gain in which a specially constructed mannekin (Kemar) that represents the characteristics of an average human is used. Kemar is used to obtain standardized measures (eg, to compare across hearing aids) while real-ear measures are used for actual patient hearing aid fittings. The increase in SPL at the eardrum provided with the hearing aid in place is called **"insertion gain."** Insertion gain reflects not only the gain of the hearing aid itself, but any loss of the ear canal resonance characteristics. An open concha and ear canal amplify the signal's high-frequency components at approximately 2500 to 3500 Hz in adults (higher in children). However, when the concha and/or ear canal are filled with an earmold or hearing aid, this high-frequency resonance may be lost. This loss of ear canal resonance is called **"insertion loss."** Because the insertion loss can vary from patient to patient, each patient's individual ear canal resonance must be measured so that the hearing aid selected will provide the gain needed to compensate for the hearing loss while also providing enough high-frequency gain to overcome any insertion loss.

Maximum Power Output (MPO)

The hearing aid's maximum power output is the aid's maximum output in response to a high-level input signal. Most patients need gain only for soft or moderate level input signals. If the hearing aid's maximum output is not kept below the patient's tolerance level, the patient will reject the hearing aid. Additionally, it is important that the hearing aid's output does not cause a noise-induced hearing loss, thus MPO levels are carefully fit, particularly in children. MPO is generally measured in the hearing aid test box using an SSPL90 (saturation sound pressure level with a 90 dB SPL input) curve. The SSPL90 curve is obtained by measuring the hearing aid's output with the volume control full-on and a 90 dB SPL input signal. The MPO measures the peak output at any one frequency, and the HFA-SSPL 90 reports the average MPO for 1000, 1600, and 2500 Hz.

Several methods are available for limiting the MPO. **Linear hearing aids** use **peak clipping**. A linear hearing aid provides essentially the same amount of gain, irrespective of input, until the hearing aid goes into saturation. When the hearing aid saturates, the peaks of the output signal are simply clipped off. This peak clipping causes substantial distortion in the hearing aid's output when it saturates. However, some of the new Class D type circuitry is linear but has lower distortion. Nonetheless, for most patients, it is preferable to use **compression** or **automatic gain control (AGC) circuitry**. The compression hearing aid's output is dependent on its input. Therefore, these hearing aids provide greater gain for low or moderate intensity signals than for high intensity signals. Compression output limiting also prevents much of the distortion for high input signals because the output is not peak clipped. There are many types of compression circuitry. For example **wide dynamic range compression (WDRC)** can provide much greater amplification for low-intensity signals than for medium-intensity signals while providing less or no gain for high-intensity signals as opposed to compression output limiting only, which provides linear amplification for low- and medium-intensity signals but controls high intensity signals with compression output limiting. The **K-AMP circuit** is a type of WDRC that provides gain and high-frequency emphasis for low-intensity signals but provides little or no gain or high-frequency emphasis for high-intensity signals. WDRC is frequently very helpful for patients with recruitment because it can help compensate for their abnormal loudness growth. WDRC often allows even patients with severe recruitment to hear a a wide intensity range of sounds comfortably. **Multiband compression** allows for different amounts of compression and output limiting for different frequency bands. Multiband compression can be very useful for patients with more recruitment at some frequencies than at others. Many other types of compression circuitry exist, but physicians may not need to be familiar with all of them.

Noise Suppression Circuitry

Many types of "noise suppression" circuitry exist. In reality, hearing aids cannot currently amplify speech alone and eliminate all background noise because speech and noise frequencies overlap. However, because most noise tends to occur at low frequencies, circuits that reduce low frequencies will usually reduce background noise relative to speech. Vowel sounds have primarily low-frequency content and consonant sounds generally have more mid- and high-frequency content. However, vowels have more energy than most consonants and therefore reducing amplification for vowels usually does not significantly reduce speech understanding and may increase it if noise is reduced to a greater degree. Most hearing-impaired individuals have the most difficulty recognizing consonant sounds because they are usually less intense and tend to comprise primarily high frequencies, a particular problem for patients with high-frequency hearing loss. Many consonants (eg, "s," "sh," "f," etc) are not voiced (the larynx does not vibrate to produce them). Therefore, their acoustic energy is limited. When low-frequency noise is reduced, these high-frequency consonants become easier to hear. Most hearing aids' frequency responses provide more gain for high frequencies than for low frequencies in all situations. However, a "low-frequency cut" to reduce low frequencies even further can be helpful in noisy situations. A hearing aid can be constantly set in the "low-frequency cut" condition, but some patients perceive the sound quality to be "harsh" or "tinny" in quiet and prefer more low-frequency energy in quiet listening situations to enhance overall quality and perception of distant sounds.

Some programmable hearing aids have multi-memory capability. These multi-memory hearing aids allow different hearing aid settings for different listening environments to be programmed into the hearing aid. The patient can then access the different settings via a remote control. Sometimes a program may be set for a specific noise environment that the patient frequently encounters (eg, car noise for a taxi driver). Some hearing aids are referred to as automatic signal processing (ASP hearing aids) or adaptive frequency response hearing aids because they adjust the hearing aid's frequency response in response to the intensity level of low frequencies in the listening environment. These circuits generally are most effective for a steady-state noise (eg, air conditioner) and may be less effective for rapidly varying noise (eg, group listening situations) or noise in the high-frequency range. Some hearing aids also have directional microphones that can be activated to reduce the microphones' sensitivity to noise from behind the patient.

HEARING AID FITTING

Great progress has been made in hearing aid fittings over the last two decades. Hearing aids are now typically fitted using **prescriptive hearing aid fittings** with **real-ear measures**. In this method, the patient's audiogram is entered into the real-ear measurement system's computer. Then a small probe microphone is placed in the patient's ear canal and the patient's ear canal resonance (**real-ear unaided response, "REUR"**) is read into the real-ear system. The audiologist then selects the desired method for computing **target gain**. Target gain is the desired amount of hearing aid gain at each frequency for that particular patient based on the audiogram and the patient's ear canal resonance measurement. Several different methods exist for computing target gain and different formulas may be used for different patients. The purpose of the various target gain formulas is to bring all speech sounds within audible range for normal and usually for soft speech. However, most hearing aid fittings for moderate or greater hearing losses are not intended to bring all hearing thresholds for all sounds within a normal range because most patients with sensorineural hearing loss also suffer from recruitment and will not readily accept that much gain.

The audiologist then orders the appropriate hearing aid to provide the desired target gain. The audiologist also selects the appropriate MPO and output limiting circuitry based on the patient's uncomfortable loudness levels and tolerance levels as well as any other special circuitry desired (eg, noise suppression, telecoil). When the hearing aid arrives, the audiologist first checks the hearing aid's electroacoustic characteristics in the hearing aid test box, and if it does not meet specifications, it is returned to the manufacturer. If the hearing aid meets specifications, the patient is tested with the small probe microphone near the tympanic membrane, with the hearing aid in place and set to desired volume (**real-ear aided response, "REAR"**). The hearing aid's output (in situ gain) is then compared to the target gain on the computer screen and adjusted until the hearing aid's output curve and target gain curve match. Although a direct match between the hearing aid's response in the wearer's ear and the target curve is not always achieved, the target presents a reasonable starting point for the fitting.

In some cases, particularly in children, additional functional gain measures may be made. Some programmable and digital hearing aids have their own target gain computation systems built into the programming device, but many audiologists still double check the output on the real-ear system.

Earmold Modifications

Earmold modifications can be used to modify the hearing aid's output. With advances in hearing aid technology employing ITE, ITC, and CIC designs that do not use earmolds, audiologists are less dependent on earmold modifications than in the past, but they can still be useful, particularly in children. As mentioned previously, a **nonoccluding or open earmold** markedly reduces low-frequency energy and may be helpful for mild high-frequency steeply sloping hearing losses or ears that require substantial ventilation. A **vent**, which is a hole in the earmold extending from the ear canal or earmold's bore to the outside, can be used to reduce a pressure sensation, the occlusion effect, or moisture build-up in the ear canal and hearing aid (especially useful for patients who have draining ears and/or TM perforations), and, depending on the type and size of vent, to reduce low-frequency amplification. A **Libby Horn** is created by hollowing out the inside of the canal portion of the earmold so that its internal diameter and associated tubing gradually increases toward the tip. The Libby Horn enhances high-frequency amplification by altering the earmold's resonance characteristics. A **"reverse horn"** has the opposite effect. **Acoustic damping material** (eg, lamb's wool) can be placed in the earmold's bore or tubing to smooth peaks in the hearing aid's frequency response but is rarely needed with newer circuitry hearing aids.

Changing the BTE earmold's tubing can alter the hearing aid's frequency response. Increasing the length or internal diameter of the tubing can shift the frequency response to slightly reduce high-frequency and increase low-frequency output. With new hearing aids, tubing modifications are rarely used to modify hearing aid output. Tubing length is simply selected to provide a good fit of the BTE over the pinna. Tubing thickness is sometimes increased for a high-gain BTE to reduce feedback. Tubing does need periodic replacement because it can become hard, discolored, or loose (particularly if the patient removes the hearing aid by pulling on the tubing).

Because ears continue to grow and change shape, children will need new earmolds about every 6 months and adults every few years to prevent feedback. For ITEs or canal aids, the hearing aid may need to be recased at similar intervals.

Hearing aids can exacerbate cerumen impaction problems or ear canal skin disorders, and the patient accordingly may need periodic medical assistance.

ADJUSTMENT TO HEARING AIDS

Even optimally fitted hearing aids will not return hearing to normal. In sensorineural hearing losses, the ear will distort signals introduced into it, and although hearing aids can render sounds audible, they may not "sound the way they used to." If hearing impaired patients do not seek amplification soon after the onset of the hearing loss, they may have forgotten how noisy the environment really is. Patients frequently complain that they do not want to hear the air conditioner, the refrigerator, and so on, but these are noises that persons with normal hearing hear all the time, and they must learn to ignore them over time. Noise suppression circuitry can reduce some background noise but cannot entirely eliminate it. In fact, one of the purposes of the hearing aid fitting is to put patients back in touch with their auditory environments.

The patients' own voices may sound strange or unpleasant to them, perhaps similar to hearing one's own voice on a tape recorder for the first time. Patients need to be reminded that they have not heard their own voice normally for a long time and a period of adjustment will be required. Patients with moderate to profound hearing losses may discover that they have been talking very loudly without hearing aids and will need to readjust their speech level.

Patients with high-frequency hearing losses may report amplified sound to be "harsh" or "tinny" when the high frequencies are restored to audible range. If the high-frequency areas of the cochlea are severely damaged, amplification may render high-frequency sounds audible but perhaps the signal is being carried on neurons coded for a different frequency region because the high-frequency hair cells and neurons in the cochlea's basal turn are no longer functional.

The term **"auditory regression"** is used when patients have forgotten sounds that they used to hear. Learning to recognize specific sounds again may take weeks or months. If patients do not consistently wear the hearing aids, they may never adjust.

If patients have difficulty adjusting to hearing aids, they should return to the audiologist to ensure that the hearing aids are working properly and to set up a program to adjust to the aids. These programs might include working with patients and their families on communication strategies or setting up hearing aid wearing schedules starting with relatively quiet listening situations and then progressing to more complex environments.

WHAT IS THE DIFFERENCE BETWEEN AN AUDIOLOGIST AND A "HEARING AID SPECIALIST"?

To obtain the Certificate of Clinical Competence in Audiology (CCC-A) from the American Speech-Language-Hearing Association, an audiologist must have at least a master's degree in audiology with nationally prescribed coursework, pass national board exams in audiology, and have a supervised fellowship year (for a minimum of 7 years of training). A doctorate in audiology requires the aforementioned credentials plus another 3 to 6 years of training. The credentials of "hearing aid specialists," "hearing aid dealers," "instrument specialists," and so on are determined individually by each state's licensure board where licensure exists. Usually only a high school education or "good moral character" is required with no formal training. Some states require the individual to pass a multiple choice test or a "hands on" test to be licensed or certified. Thus, patients should be directed to audiologists for audiologic testing and selection and fitting of hearing aids.

Always be certain that the person you refer your patients to will work with them over time to ensure that their fitting is satisfactory. Patients frequently need return visits to become skilled in handling and caring for their hearing aids. Counseling the patients and their families regarding communication skills may be critical to success. Ask how many follow-up visits are included in the purchase price and what the return policy is. Most reputable places offer a 30-day return period, and in many states, it is legally required. It is important that the clinic you refer to will still be available in the future years when your patients need service and ensure that the clinic will provide service and repairs when needed. Encourage your patients to return to the audiologist for more help if they are having trouble with their hearing aids. Many times a simple adjustment can greatly enhance patient satisfaction. Other times the patient's hearing or hearing aids may have changed and retesting will identify the problem so that it may be corrected.

Make sure that the clinic dispenses a variety of brands and types of hearing aids so that each patient can obtain an optimum fit. As discussed in *Consumer Reports* (November 1993: 716-721), hearing aids purchased from single-brand dispensers (eg, Miracle Ear), may cost twice as much for the same technology as hearing aids purchased elsewhere. If you are not already familiar with the clinic, check with the Better Business Bureau or hearing aid licensure board to determine if there is a history of patient complaints

Summary: Most hearing-impaired patients can benefit from some form of amplification. Rapid advances in technology allow hearing aids to be fitted according to each patient's hearing loss and communication needs using computerized prescriptive fitting techniques. Many circuits and options can be housed in a wide array of hearing aid styles depending on the patient's needs and preferences.

Self-Assessment Questions

1. A real estate broker with a profound sensorineural hearing loss in the left ear and a high-frequency hearing loss for 4000 Hz and above in the right ear reports difficulty in group situations. What is your advice?

2. A 2-month-old infant has absent otoacoustic emissions and ABR results suggesting severe bilateral hearing loss. When should the child be fitted with hearing aids and why?
What type of hearing aids would be appropriate?

3. A patient with bilateral familial sensorineural hearing loss has noted a relatively rapid progression of the loss in the last 2 years. What type of hearing aids would be most appropriate?

4. An 8-year-old girl has bilateral hearing aids and has performed very well with them. However, she is having trouble in her new classroom, which has some background noise and a relatively soft spoken teacher. What would you recommend?

5. When referring a patient, how can you tell if a hearing aid center is using state-of-the-art fitting methods?

Answers to Self-Assessment Questions

1. A CROS fitting with a microphone on the left ear and the signal routed to the right ear with a nonoccluding earmold on the right side should provide significant benefit to this patient. Another option would be to leave the left ear unaided and fit the right ear with a high-frequency hearing aid, probably a CIC, but this arrangement would require the patient to position the better ear near the speaker and the patient would still have trouble in group listening situations.

2. This child should be fitted with binaural hearing aids immediately to maximize speech and language acquisition and to optimize chances for normal development of the central auditory pathways. Unless the pinnae and external ears are malformed, the child would usually be fitted with small BTE hearing aids with soft earmolds.

3. Programmable hearing aids would be optimal because, as the hearing loss changes, the hearing aids can be reset to accommodate the new hearing thresholds rather than requiring the patient to pur-

chase new hearing aids each time his hearing changes. Programmable hearing aids also can usually be set to accommodate unusual audiometric configurations that may accompany familial hearing loss or other disorders (eg, meningitis, Ménière's disease).

4. This child should be fitted with an auditory trainer so that the teacher's voice can be transmitted directly to the child without interference from the background noise.

Under the Americans with Disabilities Act, the school district is obligated to provide these services when indicated. Naturally reducing the background noise, if possible, and having the school audiologist and/or speech-language pathologist counsel the teacher regarding methods for communicating with the hearing impaired would also be appropriate.

5. Be sure that the center uses real-ear measures with prescriptive hearing aid fittings and is staffed by ASHA-certified audiologists.

References and Further Reading

1. Crandell C, Smaldino J, Flexer C. *Sound Field FM Amplification.* San Diego, Calif: Singular Publishing Group Inc; 1995
2. *Consumer Reports.* "How to Buy a Hearing Aid" (1993 November): 716-721
3. Lybarger S. The physical and electroacoustic characteristics of hearing aids. In: J Katz, ed. *Handbook of Clinical Audiology.* Baltimore, Md: Williams and Wilkins; 1985:849-884.
4. Mueller G, Hawkins D, Northern J, eds. *Probe Microphone Measurements: Hearing Aid Selection and Measurements.* San Diego, Calif: Singular Publishing Group Inc; 1992.
5. Sandlin RE, ed. *Understanding Digitally Programmable Hearing Aids.* Boston, Mass: Allyn and Bacon; 1994.
6. Sandlin RE, ed. *Handbook of Hearing Aid Amplification: Theoretical and Technical Considerations.* vol 1. San Diego, Calif: Singular Publishing Group Inc; 1995
7. Sandlin RE, ed. *Handbook of Hearing Aid Amplification: Clinical Considerations and Fitting Practices.* vol 2. San Diego, Calif: Singular Publishing Group Inc; 1995.

7

Cochlear Implants and Tactile Aids

OVERVIEW: This chapter briefly reviews cochlear implants and tactile aids, which are the primary device options for bilaterally profoundly deaf individuals who cannot benefit from traditional hearing aids. Because most physicians will not be directly involved with these types of devices, less detail is provided than in the chapter on hearing aids. Instead physicians are provided with a brief description of the devices, candidacy criteria, realistic performance expectations, cost and time considerations, and suggestions for choosing a cochlear implant referral center.

COCHLEAR IMPLANTS

The Device

Cochlear implants consist of a microphone that picks up acoustic stimuli and transduces them into electrical signals, a **speech processor** (which currently looks like a body style hearing aid) with an output wire that connects to an **external coil** (outside the head), which transmits the signal across the skull to an implanted **internal coil** (inside the head), which in turn sends the signal to an electrode, or series of electrodes, that are usually implanted into the scala tympani of the cochlea. Electrodes can be placed on or near the round window if they cannot be placed intracochlearly (eg, due to a completely ossified cochlea), but this is unusual. For individuals with severed VIIIth nerves (eg, postsurgical bilateral vestibular Schwannoma, as in acoustic neuroma patients having Neurofibromatosis II), an implant can be placed on the cochlear nucleus, in which case it is called an **auditory brainstem implant**. The external coil rests over the internal coil in the mastoid and typically stays in place by a magnetic pull between the external and internal coils. In the past, percutaneous plugs were used with a hardwire plug extending through the skull. Although this arrangement has been helpful for research, it has been largely discontinued because of localized tissue reactions and aesthetics. A microphone is generally placed on an earmold or behind-the-ear hearing aid casing to receive sound in a normal location.

Although much early research and implantation involved the use of single channel, single electrode devices (eg, the House implant), multichannel devices are generally used today. Each electrode or pair of electrodes can then stimulate a certain area of the cochlea, thus providing some frequency specificity. Naturally, even 22 electrode pairs cannot provide the frequency specificity of over 30,000 individual VIIIth nerve neurons, but they can provide useful information. The placement of the stimulated electrodes, the voltage level delivered to the electrodes, the stimulation rate, pulse duration, timing strategies, the transitions from one signal delivery to the next, and the various methods of pairing the electrodes can all be varied to help patients identify and distinguish among different sounds.

The process of setting all of these parameters for a given patient once the implant is in place is called **mapping**. Minimally, mapping includes setting (for each electrode or electrode pair) the audible threshold; the maximum output level based on tolerance levels, loudness growth, loudness balancing across electrodes; frequency mapping (which speech frequencies stimulate which electrodes, usually based on pitch matching); inactivating electrodes that, when stimulated, cause pain or other unpleasant sensations; and a host of other factors that may be specific to the implant's particular processing strategy.

A cochlear implant's **processing strategy** determines how its speech processor analyzes incoming sound and converts it to electrical stimulation. For example, only certain aspects of speech may be detected and converted to stimulation (feature detection) or an analogue version of the entire signal may be processed and delivered. Development of processing strategies is a continuing area of research, and it is anticipated that most major advances in cochlear implant technology over the next few years will involve the speech processors. They will become smaller and will probably become available in an ear-level model, appearing similar to a behind-the-ear hearing aid. Speech processing strategies have markedly improved over the last decade, but will further improve, and may include flexible processing strategies that change as the listening environment changes.

Although not all physicians will be directly involved with patients who need cochlear implants, they should be aware of when and where to refer such patients. The audiologists and otolaryngologists directly involved in cochlear implant programs must allocate significant time to keeping current with advances in this technology.

It should be emphasized, however, that the biggest time commitment on the part of the patient and the cochlear implant center is to the rehabilitation program in which the patient will learn to use the device and to recognize and interpret the stimulation provided by the cochlear implant. Patients and physicians often tend to focus on the surgical implantation and device mapping, which constitute only a relatively small part of the overall process (especially for children).

SELECTION OF CANDIDATES FOR COCHLEAR IMPLANTS

Profoundly deafened patients who have tried hearing aids without measurable benefit (usually not even sound detection) for normal conversational level speech may be candidates for cochlear implants. Criteria for implantation are changing, and there are plans to develop cochlear implants for partially hearing-impaired individuals; however, currently, candidates for cochlear implants must have bilateral, profound, sensorineural hearing loss. Children usually must be at least 2 years old and adults should have become deaf after they developed some speech and language (postlingually deaf). Some prelingually deafened adults have been implanted but generally with less than optimal results. Even postlingually deafened adults usually have much better outcomes if they had hearing at least through the age of 6 years.

Some professionals believe that children should be implanted prior to 2 years of age because the central auditory pathways may not fully develop if they are not stimulated at a very early age. Others argue that we need to wait until we have more complete behavioral audiologic information, including hearing aid performance, to ensure that we do not implant a child who could perform better with hearing aids. Additionally, head growth with the implant in place and children's propensity for otitis media are all considerations. However, data show that prelingually deafened children first implanted after age 6 years rarely have good success with cochlear implants, which suggests that there is a "window" for optimal implantation. Current FDA regulations require that the child be at least 2 years of age, although in the future the required age is expected to drop.

Many medical, psychological, and social factors need to be considered in determining cochlear implant candidacy. Usually cochlear implant patients should have no other disabling condition (eg, blindness, mental retardation, severe emotional disturbance or behavioral problems, or an unstable home environment), although some programs will make exceptions on an individual basis. Additionally, children must be in an environment that provides abundant auditory stimulation. Malformed cochleae or prior meningitis with bony growth in the cochlea may be problematic for implantation. Other medical contraindications (eg, chronic otitis media) may also preclude or delay implantation.

As previously mentioned, surgically placing the electrodes in the cochlea is only a small part of the total cochlear implant rehabilitation process. Cochlear implant mapping strategies and rehabilitation programs vary from clinic to clinic, but are generally quite extensive. First, the patient must simply develop sound awareness with the implant and then hopefully progress to gross and then fine discrimination among different sounds. Many patients can then work toward closed-set (multiple choice) and open-set sound recognition and then to comprehension; however, not all patients will be able to perform these tasks even with intensive rehabilitation programs. Realistic expectations and ongoing counseling are essential for all patients. If a patient's expectations are too high, the cochlear implant may be rejected out of frustration and the patient may feel a sense of betrayal.

In postlingually deafened adults, intensive aural rehabilitation may last only a couple of months, followed by less intensive aural rehabilitation therapy and annual follow-up visits. Their rehabilitation program usually includes instruction on using the cochlear implant, auditory training, and instruction on structuring the listening environment. Family members will be included in the aural rehabilitation process, particularly for developing communication strategies. A home program for the patient and family may be recommended. Because postlingually deafened adults generally acquired good speech and language skills before deafness and because they usually can remember hearing speech sounds, they generally will progress more rapidly than prelingually deafened patients. Prelingually deafened adults are not as commonly implanted and need special and intensive rehabilitation programs because they have never heard auditory stimuli and did not acquire speech and language through auditory channels. They may or may not adapt successfully to the implant.

Particularly for children, the speech and language therapy and auditory training will be extensive and ongoing, probably to adulthood, with a goal of constant improvement. Even in adulthood, annual visits will always be required. Just mapping the electrodes, particularly in a child, may require several visits over a period of months. As the child becomes a better listener over the years, more sophisticated mapping may be done. Additionally, new hardware and software is constantly being developed and each new development may require the patient to return to the clinic for upgrades. The child's aural rehabilitation program may include all of the components of the adult's program, but modified for the child's age. Because most implanted children will have no memory of hearing speech, the auditory training will be slower and more extensive. The child's rehabilitation program also will include heavy parental involvement. Because the child must still acquire speech and language, much of the therapy will address this goal. At home, everyday activities can be turned into opportunities for developing auditory and speech and language skills. Therefore, the adult patient, or the child and his or her family, must be highly motivated, have appropriate expectations, and be willing and able to commit the time and effort involved. Similarly, school personnel need to be counseled regarding the cochlear implant and integrating the child into the educational environment.

Finances, not only for the implant itself, but also for the rehabilitation program, should be fully discussed with the patient and family. Even when insurance pays for the implant, it may not cover the rehabilitation program. As discussed by Tye-Murray (1993), the total cost of the formal evaluations, hospitalization, surgery, the device itself, and the fitting may be $35,000. The follow-up visits and rehabilitation program are not included in that figure.

Physicians should also be aware that there are many cultural issues involved in implanting deaf individuals. Many members of the deaf community do not view deafness as a disability, but rather as a cultural difference. Consequently, these individuals may be openly opposed to cochlear implants for themselves or their children.

EXPECTED BENEFITS FROM
COCHLEAR IMPLANTS

The amount of benefit for a given patient cannot be adequately predicted prior to implantation. The etiology of the hearing loss, number of surviving auditory neurons, number of years since deafness onset, and a host of other factors will influence success; nonetheless the patient's postimplantation functional level cannot be known in advance. Most individuals will receive sound awareness, some environmental sound recognition, and speechreading enhancement. Most audiologists advise their patients that anything more is considered a "bonus." Individuals with speech impairments secondary to their hearing loss may experience improved speech production. Many individuals will have improved pattern perception and word recognition. Some "stars" have excellent open-set word recognition and can even converse on the telephone. Although the "stars" are frequently featured in promotions for cochlear implants and are very encouraging, patients must understand that not every patient will receive such excellent benefit. In adults, most improvement occurs in the first 9 months. In children, slow improvement in benefit is usually obtained over a period of years following implantation.

Promotions for children's cochlear implants often show a wide-eyed, delighted child hearing sound for the first time. In reality, many children are not initially delighted with the stimulation provided by the implant and demonstrable benefits may not be seen until 12 to 18 months postimplantation. These results are to be expected if the child's "hearing age" is considered (ie, the normal infant has been hearing not only from birth but for several months before birth and still needs several months before consistently demonstrating responses to auditory stimuli). The congenitally deaf child similarly will need time to acquire auditory skills.

The only individuals who truly know what a cochlear implant sounds like are cochlear implant users. However postlingually deafened adults have described speech as sounding like a poor quality, mechanical, cartoonlike, voice, often described as a "duck." Nonetheless, even a poor quality signal can be a significant improvement over total silence.

TACTILE AIDS

Patients should have an opportunity to try tactile aids before considering a cochlear implant or when a cochlear implant is inappropriate for them. A wide variety of vibro- and electro-tactile aids has been used and developed over the years. A simple tactile aid consists of a microphone, a processor, and a signal delivery system (eg, electrodes or vibrators). Multichannel stimulators are larger but allow a larger area to be stimulated across different frequencies to improve discrimination among frequencies. Tactile aids usually stimulate the hand, waist, wrist, forearm, neck, forehead, or most commonly the sternum.

Although some tactile aids have been found to provide speechreading improvement, none has been as successful as cochlear implants, and no tactile aid user has been able to carry on a conversation relying solely on the input from a tactile aid. Tactile aids can help patients identify and discriminate sounds and may improve speechreading. They can also be used in conjunction with hearing aids. Even more than with cochlear implants, tactile aid fitting requires a training/rehabilitation program to be successful.

Tactile aids do not require surgery and do not destroy any cochlear structures. Therefore, tactile aids may be appropriate for individuals in whom cochlear implants are contraindicated (eg, chronic otitis media, absent or malformed cochleae) or in individuals who want to wait until cochlear implants are further improved. Research in tactile aids is continuing and perhaps new future advances will bring better results.

SELECTING A COCHLEAR IMPLANT CENTER

Physicians should carefully select the cochlear implant center to which they refer patients. Some centers use only one type of implant; others have a selection of types from which to choose. Some centers see a restricted range of patients; others may have programs encompassing a wide range of ages and concomitant disabilities. Physicians should be sure that the center has a complete cochlear implant team including diagnostic and rehabilitation audiologists, speech-language pathologists, otolaryngologists (usually pediatric and/or neuro-otologists), and psychologists.

For new programs, physicians should also be certain that adequate staff time has been allowed for the mapping and rehabilitation programs and that the center has the financial base to support these programs. Time must also be allotted for the rehabilitation audiologist to work with the schools because many schools will need assistance in fully accommodating the child with an implant. Additionally, there should be more than one audiologist fully skilled and constantly current in the mapping and rehabilitation programs to ensure that service will always be available for the patient.

Some centers have started cochlear implant programs, only to close them because they were not prepared for the extensive financial and time commitment required to establish and maintain the rehabilitation programs and to remain current in new techniques, including software and hardware upgrades. This situation leaves patients in the unfortunate position of trying to find a center for follow-up. Many programs are relatively unwilling to assume the follow-up for patients they have not implanted. The actual implantation is generally lucrative, but the rehabilitation and follow-up services frequently are not. Patients may also have trouble finding a new center close to home that carries their particular kind of implant.

Because cochlear implants are rapidly developing, a clinic must have a substantial cochlear implant patient base to justify investing the staff time to develop and maintain adequate expertise in this rapidly changing area and be prepared to handle the variety of patient problems that may develop. If only a few patients per year are implanted, the program probably will not be able to justify the time and financial investments in software and hardware upgrades for state-of-the-art service.

Additionally, a cochlear implant program should offer a wide array of other options for deaf individuals, including assistive devices, tactile aids, and a strong emphasis on aural rehabilitation programs. An excellent hearing aid program should also be available at the center. Some patients, when provided with optimal hearing aid fittings, are no longer candidates for cochlear implants.

These considerations are not intended to discourage physicians from referring patients for cochlear implants. For deaf individuals who cannot benefit from hearing aids, cochlear implants can frequently return them to the hearing world and, in some cases, the change is remarkable.

Summary: Cochlear implants can be very helpful for patients with profound bilateral hearing loss that cannot obtain measurable benefit from hearing aids for normal conversational level speech. However, patient performance with cochlear implants cannot be completely predicted in advance. The rapid development of cochlear implant technology in this area will not only improve patients' speech perception but may also expand the range of patient eligibility by reducing the allowable age for implantation and the degrees of hearing loss that can be fit. Further these devices are being miniaturized for better cosmetic appeal. However, an excellent aural rehabilitation program is critical to the patient's success with the cochlear implant and should be a major, if not the major consideration in selecting a program. Tactile aids may also be useful for some patients, particularly if they are not eligible for a cochlear implant.

Self-Assessment Questions

1. Which professionals are required for a cochlear implant team?

2. List the components of a cochlear implant.

3. List three reasons why a patient may not be eligible for a cochlear implant.

4. A patient with Neurofibromatosis Type II has had bilateral vestibular Schwannoma removal. What options are available to this patient?

Answers to Self-Assessment Questions

1. The team should include diagnostic and rehabilitation audiologists, speech-language pathologists, otolaryngologists (usually pediatric and/or neuro-otologists), and psychologists.

2. Cochlear implant components include a microphone, a speech processor, an external coil, an internal coil, and the stimulating electrodes.

3. The prelingually deafened adult or the child under 2 years of age may not be eligible. If patients have less than profound hearing loss or receive significant benefit from hearing aids, they are not candidates. Medical contraindications may include chronic otitis media, malformed, bone-filled, or absent cochleae. In some cases patients with medical contraindications may be fitted with implants. For example, the bone-filled cochlea may be drilled out or the patient may be fitted with electrodes placed on or near the round window, but performance prognosis is reduced. Psychological, behavioral, motivational, family, and financial problems can all be factors in determining candidacy for cochlear implantation.

4. This patient may be a candidate for a brainstem implant, which is available only at selected cochlear implant centers. If the patient does not want or is not eligible for a brainstem implant, a referral to one of these centers would still be appropriate because they can advise the patient regarding tactile aids, assistive listening devices, and other rehabilitation programs including communication strategies, speechreading, and sign language. A counseling program with a psychologist skilled in the area could also be very helpful to this patient and his or her family.

References and Further Reading

1. Cooper H, ed. *Cochlear Implants: A Practical Guide.* San Diego, Calif: Singular Publishing Group Inc; 1991.
2. Mecklenburg D. Cochlear implants and rehabilitative processes. In: Sandlin R, ed. *Handbook of Hearing Aid Amplification: Theoretical and Technical Considerations.* vol II. San Diego, Calif: Singular Publishing Group Inc; 1995.
3. Nevins ME, Chute PM. *Children with Cochlear Implants in Educational Settings.* San Diego, Calif: Singular Publishing Group Inc; 1996.
4. Oller DK, ed. Tactile aids for the hearing impaired. *Sem Hearing.* 1995;16:4
5. Shallop JS, Mecklenburg DJ. Technical aspects of cochlear implants. In: Sandlin R, ed. *Handbook of Hearing Aid Amplification: Theoretical and Technical Considerations.* vol 1. San Diego, Calif: Singular Publishing Group Inc: 1995.
6. Tye-Murray N. Aural rehabilitation and patient management. In: Tyler RS, ed. *Cochlear Implants: Audiological Foundations.* San Diego, Calif: Singular Publishing Group Inc; 1993.
7. Tyler RS, ed. *Cochlear Implants: Audiological Foundations.* San Diego, Calif: Singular Publishing Group Inc; 1993.

8

Site of Lesion Testing

OVERVIEW: This chapter reviews many of the traditional site-of-lesion tests in audiology including the short increment sensitivity index, Bekesy audiometry, loudness balance tests, tone decay, and acoustic reflex decay. Many of the most powerful site-of-lesion tests including tympanometry for middle ear function, acoustic reflex testing for a variety of lesions, otoacoustic emissions for cochlear function, and electrophysiologic measures for detection of retrocochlear disorders are discussed in separate Chapters 2, 4, and 5. The audiologic basic battery, described in Chapter 1, is always the starting point for any diagnostic audiologic workup and provides important information about the probable site-of-lesion underlying the hearing loss.

TRADITIONAL AUDIOLOGIC SITE-OF-LESION TESTS

An VIIIth nerve lesion usually is suspected when a patient has a uni-lateral or asymmetric, sensorineural hearing loss, particularly when the hearing loss is accompanied by poor word recognition and/or tin-nitus. Historically, the following tests have been used primarily to dif-ferentiate between cochlear and retrocochlear (VIIIth nerve) sites of lesion. As otoacoustic emissions developed to assess cochlear function and electrophysiologic measures and radiographic imaging improved to assess retrocochlear pathways, the traditional tests covered in this chapter have largely fallen into disuse because their sensitivity and specificity are not as high as the newer tests and because they require careful patient attention to the listening task, whereas otoacoustic emissions and electrophysiologic measures generally do not. However these tests can still be useful for certain applications, and physicians should be aware of them. Other psychophysical measures for site-of-lesion testing exist but are not included here because they have never been commonly used in clinical practice.

The Short Increment Sensitivity Index (SISI)

Classically, the SISI test consists of a high-frequency pure tone pre-sented to the patient's ear at 20 dB SL via earphone. At 5 second inter-vals, the tone momentarily increases in intensity and then returns to the baseline level. Each time patients detect the intensity change, they push the response button to notify the audiologist that the change was detected. The size of the intensity change is gradually decreased from 5 to 1 dB. Then, 20 intervals containing the 1 dB intensity change are presented and the number of changes the patient detects is recorded and converted to a percentage score. Generally, scores of 70% or greater are considered indicative of cochlear disorder and scores below 70% are considered as not indicative of cochlear disorder (ie, either normal or retrocochlear lesion). Some consider scores of 80% or above as "highly indicative" and scores of 20% or below "nonindicative" of cochlear disorder, with scores between those two ranges relatively nondiagnostic.

In some cases, a high intensity level (eg, 75 dB HL) SISI may be performed. This test is administered in basically the same manner as the classic SISI test, but at this high intensity level, usually both nor-mals and patients with cochlear disorder can detect the 1 dB increment while patients with retrocochlear lesions (eg, VIIIth nerve tumor) gen-erally cannot.

Thus, by using a combination of low-level and high-level SISI tests, the clinician can generally distinguish between normals (who usually cannot detect the 1 dB increment on the low-intensity test but can on the high-intensity test), patients with cochlear disorder (who generally can detect the 1 dB increment on both tests if they have moderate or greater sensorineural hearing losses), and patients with retrocochlear lesion (who usually cannot detect the 1 dB increment on either test). Physicians should recall, however, that acoustic neuromas can compromise cochlear blood supply and thus yield cochlear symptoms. Additionally, patients with mild sensorineural hearing losses of cochlear origin may yield normal findings.

The sensitivity and specificity of SISI tests for site-of-lesion testing are lower than more recently developed measures. Since the development of otoacoustic emissions (which provide an excellent, objective, measure of cochlear function) and electrophysiologic assessments and improved radiographic imaging (which detect retrocochlear disorders), the SISI is no longer commonly used for discriminating between cochlear and retrocochlear site of lesion, but is occasionally used as part of a test battery. There are many reports of positive SISI test results in the presence of VIIIth nerve lesions, and several authors have recommended against the use of SISI for differentiating between cochlear and retrocochlear hearing loss. Additionally, the sensitivity of the SISI to cochlear hearing loss is very dependent on the degree of hearing loss. Normal findings may be obtained in cases of mild cochlear hearing loss, but positive cochlear findings will generally be obtained in cases of cochlear hearing loss of a moderate or greater degree.

Some clinicians have assumed that the ability to detect the 1 dB increments on the classic SISI reflects recruitment because normally hearing individuals cannot detect such a small intensity change. However, careful studies have demonstrated that the SISI is not a valid measure of recruitment. Better methods to measure recruitment exist.

Bekesy Audiometry

Bekesy audiometry used to be a standard diagnostic test for differentiating among cochlear, retrocochlear, and functional hearing losses. However, as discussed in the section on SISI testing, the advent of more accurate and objective tests has largely supplanted these earlier behavioral site-of-lesion tests. Nonetheless, the physician should be aware of Bekesy audiometry and its interpretation in order to understand behavioral correlates of various pathologies and to assist in interpreting earlier literature on otologic pathologies.

In Bekesy audiometry, a pure tone is presented to the patient through an earphone. The pure tone may be of a single or "fixed" frequency or may slowly "sweep" across frequencies, classically from low to high frequencies. Patients are instructed to push the response button when they hear the tone, whereupon the tone decreases in intensity, and to release the button when the tone is no longer heard, whereupon the tone increases in intensity. The response button and attenuator are connected to a plotter that traces patients' responses on a form similar to an audiogram.

Two traces are obtained for each stimulus type (ie, sweep or fixed frequency), one for a continuously presented stimulus ("continuous stimulus" or "C tone") and the other for a stimulus that pulses on and off ("interrupted stimulus" or "I tone"). Not only do the traces provide information about the patients' thresholds (similar to "automatic audiometry" sometimes used in industrial settings) but comparing the traces for the two stimulus types yields five distinct pattern types that can be useful in differential diagnosis.

Type I

In type I recordings, the I and C tracings overlap across the sweep frequency range. Type I recordings were considered to be indicative of normal hearing or conductive hearing loss. However, they were also sometimes seen in cases of cochlear and retrocochlear disorder.

Type II

In Type II recordings, the C trace drops approximately 10 to 20 dB below the I trace for high frequencies (generally above 1000 Hz) for the sweep frequency mode. This pattern was considered to be indicative of cochlear hearing loss, but sometimes occurred in cases of retrocochlear hearing loss.

Type III

In type III recordings, the C trace markedly drops (usually over 40 dB and often to the equipment limits) below the I trace for both fixed and sweep frequency traces. For sweep frequency traces, the C trace drops frequently below the I trace even at low frequencies and the disparity between traces usually increases as frequency is increased, but this may be more a function of time than frequency. A Type III Bekesy trace was considered to be indicative of retrocochlear hearing loss, particularly acoustic neuroma. Patients frequently have trouble perceiving a continuous tone over a period of time as reflected on this test and also on the tone decay test (see following section) and the acoustic reflex decay test (see Chapter 2, Immittance Audiometry).

Type IV

In type IV recordings, The C trace drops below the I trace across the sweep frequency range. Although the separation generally exceeds 25 dB, the C trace does not drop to the equipment limits as in Type III. A Type IV trace was considered to be indicative of retrocochlear lesion (eg, VIIIth nerve tumors).

Type V

In type V recordings, the I trace drops below the C trace across the frequency range for sweep-frequency stimuli and over time for fixed-frequency stimulation. A type V Bekesy trace is both sensitive and specific for functional (feigned) hearing loss. A person attempting to feign hearing loss will not respond until a signal is at a suprathreshold level. At suprathreshold levels, continuous stimuli are perceived as louder than interrupted stimuli of the same intensity. Therefore, a person attempting to feign hearing loss will attempt to match equal loudness for the two stimulus types and thus provide responses at lower intensities for the continuous stimulus than for the interrupted stimulus. For all other Bekesy pattern types, the I and C traces overlap or the C trace falls below the I trace. Consequently, the type V pattern is readily differentiated from other Bekesy recordings.

Diagnostic Accuracy of Bekesy Recordings

Virtually all patients with normal hearing or conductive disorder yielded a type I Bekesy. However, the Bekesy test was rarely needed for those patients. Of patients with purely cochlear disorder, almost all, depending on the study, yielded a type I or II Bekesy pattern. Of patients with acoustic neuromas or sudden hearing loss, usually about one-half to three-quarters would yield either a Type III or IV tracing with the rest yielding a Type I or II. For acoustic neuromas, as would be expected, the sensitivity was better for larger than for smaller tumors. Although Bekesy audiometry has been supplanted by superior site-of-lesion diagnostic methods, including immittance measures, otoacoustic emissions, auditory brainstem response testing, and improved radiographic techniques, it did provide useful information before the newer techniques were developed. Bekesy audiometry, like the SISI test, was always used as a part of a test battery approach including a comprehensive basic battery, acoustic reflex testing, PI-PB functions, and usually a variety of other tests.

Bekesy audiometry equipment is no longer marketed because it has been replaced by better site-of-lesion test methods. Unfortunately, Bekesy audiometry is no longer available for evaluating possible functional hearing impairment which would still be a very useful application. Sensitivity and specificity of Bekesy audiometry for feigned or exaggerated hearing loss were generally high.

Several modifications to Bekesy procedures were developed, but because Bekesy audiometry is no longer used clinically, most physicians only need to be aware of classic procedures and findings. For a more complete discussion of Bekesy audiometry and more detailed references, the reader is referred to Brunt.

Loudness Balance Tests

Loudness balance tests measure recruitment. As discussed in Chapter 1, Basic Audiologic Assessment, **recruitment** is an abnormal increase in loudness growth and is associated with cochlear disorder. For example, a patient with unilateral Ménière's disease may have a 2000 Hz hearing threshold of 45 dB HL in the affected ear and 10 dB HL in the normal ear, but an 85 dB HL signal may be perceived as equally loud in both ears although it is at a sensation level (SL) of 40 dB in the affected ear and 75 dB in the normal ear. Similarly, a patient with noise-induced hearing loss may have a threshold of 10 dB HL at 500 Hz and 50 dB HL at 2000 Hz, but at 90 dB HL both frequencies may be perceived as equally loud because recruitment is present for the high-frequency range where cochlear hearing loss has occurred.

Alternate Binaural Loudness Balance Test (ABLB)

The ABLB is used to measure recruitment when the patient has a unilateral sensorineural hearing loss. The ABLB was commonly used in differential diagnosis, but has been superseded by better diagnostic tests as previously discussed.

In the ABLB, brief tones of the same frequency are alternately presented to the two ears. Usually a stimulus frequency in the 1000 Hz to 4000 Hz range is employed because most patients, particularly those with high-frequency cochlear hearing loss, exhibit the greatest amount of recruitment in that range. The patient's task is to compare the loudness of the tone presented to the "reference ear" (the ear receiving tones of constant intensity) to the "variable ear" (the ear receiving tones of varying intensity.) The intensity of the tone in the variable ear is then adjusted until the patient perceives that it is equally loud to the tone in the reference ear. This procedure is then repeated for several reference ear intensities. The points at which signals in the reference ear and variable ear are loudness matched are then graphed in "laddergram" or chart ("loudness growth") format (see Fig 8–1).

Results of the ABLB can be categorized as complete recruitment, incomplete or partial recruitment, no recruitment, or decruitment. The classification of findings in asymmetric hearing loss is based primarily on the loudness match for high-intensity signals in the reference ear.

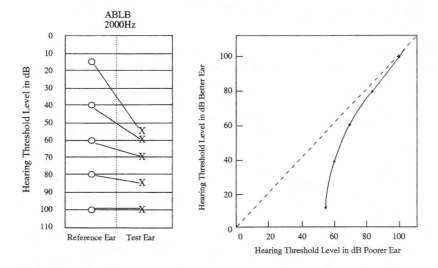

Fig 8–1. — Examples of ABLB results for a patient with complete recruitment. Results are charted as a laddergram (left) and as a loudness growth function (right).

In **complete recruitment**, a high-intensity tone is perceived as being equally loud in both ears although the thresholds are substantially different. Thus, there is **abnormal loudness growth**, which is the definition of recruitment.

In **incomplete recruitment**, high-intensity signals in the normal ear are loudness matched to signals of lesser intensity in the poorer ear, however the disparity is not as great as the asymmetry in threshold would predict. For example, a patient with 10 dB HL and 40 dB HL thresholds for 2000 Hz in the normal and poorer ear, respectively, might loudness match a 70 dB HL signal in the normal ear with an 80 dB signal in the poorer ear. Because a greater intensity signal (80 dB HL) is required in the poorer ear to be perceived as equally loud to the high level signal (70 dB) in the normal ear, complete recruitment has not occurred. However, the disparity between the two ears at threshold is 30 dB, and at a high intensity level, only 10 dB, so abnormal loudness growth and incomplete recruitment has occurred. If the same patient had **no recruitment**, the 70 dB HL signal in the normal ear would loudness match to a 100 dB HL signal in the poorer ear and thus the growth of loudness would be normal. In **decruitment**, loudness growth is abnormally decreased. Therefore, if the same patient had decruitment, the 70 dB HL signal in the normal ear would be loudness matched to a signal greater than 100 dB HL, or would not be matched at equipment limits suggesting that loudness grew more slowly in the poorer ear than in the normal ear which is suggestive of retrocochlear lesion.

Monaural Loudness Balance Test (MLB)

The MLB is similar to the ABLB, but rather than comparing loudness between ears for a single frequency, the MLB compares loudness between frequencies within a given ear. The MLB is used when the patient has symmetric, bilateral sensorineural hearing loss or only has one "dead ear" and one ear with sensorineural hearing loss. For example, for a patient with high-frequency sensorineural hearing loss, the growth of loudness at 500 Hz, where the hearing is normal, may be compared with 4000 Hz where significant hearing loss exists. The MLB does actually measure recruitment and the results are interpreted in a similar fashion as the ABLB; however, the results must be compared to equal-loudness functions for normal ears, which makes interpretation cumbersome.

Complete and incomplete recruitment suggest cochlear abnormality. No recruitment suggests cochlear normalcy, as in unilateral conductive hearing loss. Decruitment suggests retrocochlear abnormality (eg, VIIIth nerve tumors), although VIIIth nerve tumors can also cause cochlear abnormalities (ie, interruption of cochlear blood supply) and thus yield cochlear signs as well.

Sometimes recruitment tests are also used for hearing aid fittings but clinicians usually will test the uncomfortable loudness level and measure the dynamic range for those applications (see Chapter 1, The Basic Audiologic Assessment, and Chapter 6, Hearing Aids). Additionally, some programmable hearing aid manufacturers have developed loudness growth and recruitment tests to optimize programming of their hearing aids for individual patients.

Diagnostic Accuracy of Loudness Balance Testing

The ABLB and MLB are excellent tests of recruitment. Generally over three-quarters of patients with purely cochlear hearing loss will show complete or partial recruitment. Decruitment or no recruitment in conjunction with sensorineural hearing loss is considered a sign of retrocochlear disorder (eg, VIIIth nerve tumors), but the reported sensitivity and specificity of these measures for that application vary widely across studies. Up to one-quarter of cochlear hearing loss cases will demonstrate no recruitment although decruitment in those cases is rarely seen. However, VIIIth nerve tumors can cause cochlear damage and thus cochlear signs, which may account for some of the variability in diagnostic accuracy reported across studies. These tests have been replaced by better site-of-lesion tests, including otoacoustic emissions for cochlear function and electrophysiologic and radiographic measures for retrocochlear function, but remain excellent tests of recruitment and loudness growth. They are more time consuming to administer than the SISI but, unlike the SISI, actually measure recruitment.

Tone Decay Tests

If a continuous pure-tone signal is presented to the listener at a near-threshold level, eventually the signal will seem to decrease or disappear. This adaptation is called **tone decay** and occurs even in normals. However, in the presence of retrocochlear lesions, (including but not restricted to VIIIth nerve tumors), the tone generally adapts more quickly and to a greater degree. Normals can generally hear a pure tone at 20 dB SL for at least 60 seconds, but a patient with an VIIIth nerve tumor often hears a 20 dB SL tone for only a few seconds, and if the stimulus intensity is raised, usually adaptation again occurs. The amount of tone decay is the amount of threshold shift observed for that stimulus, usually within a set time frame (ie, 30 dB of tone decay in 60 seconds would mean that the tone had to be elevated to 30 dB above the patient's threshold for that frequency within a 60-second period). Some tone decay tests monitor not only the patient's ability to hear the tone, but whether there is any change in the "tonality" of the signal.

Several variations in tone decay test procedures exist. Although most variations of tone decay tests use stimuli at or near the patient's threshold for the stimulus, the Suprathreshold Adaptation Test (STAT) evaluates tone decay using very high level stimuli (eg, 110 dB SPL). Regardless of procedure, the greater the amount of tone decay, the greater the likelihood of an VIIIth nerve lesion. For example, a patient with 20 dB of tone decay would have a relatively low index of suspicion and a patient with 35 dB of tone decay would have a relatively high index of suspicion for VIIIth nerve lesion.

Diagnostic Accuracy of Tone Decay Testing

Of the behavioral site of lesion measures, tone decay and reflex measures seem to have the highest sensitivity and specificity. The biggest problem with tone decay is that its sensitivity to VIIIth nerve lesions (averaging across studies) is approximately 80% as opposed to the ABR (see Chapter 5, Electrophysiologic Measures) which has sensitivity of over 90% (average across studies approximately 95%). However, sometimes when the patient's high-frequency thresholds are so poor so as to preclude clear ABR recordings, tone decay testing can still be performed. Tone decay testing is also quick and inexpensive. If tone decay is present, certainly the possibility of a retrocochlear lesion needs to be pursued. But approximately 20% of patients with VIIIth nerve tumors will not exhibit tone decay (ie, the specificity is approximately 80% or conversely the false positive rate is approximately 20%).

Acoustic Reflexes and Acoustic Reflex Decay Testing

As discussed in Chapter 2 on immittance audiometry, in the presence of a retrocochlear lesion (eg, VIIIth nerve lesion), acoustic reflexes may be absent. If acoustic reflexes are present, acoustic reflex decay may be present. To test for **acoustic reflex decay**, a signal 10 dB above the patient's acoustic reflex threshold at either 500 Hz or 1000 Hz is presented to the ear for 10 seconds and the crossed reflex is monitored. If the amplitude of the response decreases more than 50% during the 10 second interval, it is considered to be abnormal and indicative of VIIIth nerve disorder. Frequencies above 1000 Hz are not used for acoustic reflex decay because decay at high frequencies occurs even in normal subjects. Acoustic reflex testing (including acoustic reflex decay) is neither as sensitive nor as specific as the auditory brainstem response (ABR) for detecting VIIIth nerve tumors; however, it is faster, and cheaper, which makes it a good starting point in the test battery. As discussed in Chapter 2 on immittance audiometry, acoustic reflex testing can be used to test for a wide variety of lesions, and acoustic reflex thresholds are also dependent on the type and degree of hearing loss.

Diagnostic Accuracy of Acoustic Reflex Testing

The diagnostic accuracy of acoustic reflex testing, particularly acoustic reflex decay, is seemingly slightly better than for tone decay. Most studies report slightly over 80% sensitivity in the detection of VIIIth nerve tumors, which is substantially less than ABR. The specificity is approximately 80% (or conversely the false positive rate is approximately 20%).

Performance-Intensity Functions (PI Functions or PIPB Functions)

As discussed in Chapter 1, PI functions are constructed from testing word recognition at several different intensity levels. This test can serve several purposes. From the PI function the **PB max**, or the intensity level providing the best word recognition score for phonetically balanced word lists, can be determined. The PI function can also be used as a site-of-lesion test by determining if **rollover**, a worsening of the word recognition score, occurs at high intensities. In conductive or cochlear loss, word recognition scores should continue to improve or remain the same as stimulus intensity increases. In retrocochlear lesions, (eg, VIIIth nerve tumors), scores may reach a maximum and then deteriorate.

PI functions may be time intensive and patients may become bored repeating word lists at several different levels. Further, the sensitivity and specificity for rollover is not as clearly established as for some of the other psychophysical tests. How much rollover constitutes "significant rollover" or which word lists should be used are issues that are not fully resolved. If the patient has moderate or greater hearing loss, the range over which a PI function can be tested will be limited. However, rollover on the PI function can be sensitive not only to VIIIth nerve lesion but also to brainstem and even cortical abnormalities.

Summary: None of the aforementioned tests is as sensitive as the ABR for detection of retrocochlear lesions (eg, VIIIth nerve tumors). The ABR has over 90% sensitivity (averaged across studies approximately 95%) and 80 to 90% specificity (10 to 20% false alarm rate), whereas even the best psychophysical measure has slightly over 80% sensitivity and 80% specificity. The sensitivity, even for the ABR, increases with tumor size. Because acoustic neuromas (more properly called vestibular Schwannomas) usually arise from the superior vestibular nerve, in the early stages no auditory effects may be apparent. Small intracanalicular tumors may be missed by even the ABR. Therefore, some physicians may not seek additional audiologic site-of-lesion tests when a retrocochlear lesion is suspected and instead immediately look to MRI and CT scans. However, these tests can be useful in certain instances and physicians should be aware of them and their potential roles in the differential diagnostic site-of-lesion test battery.

Self-Assessment Questions

1. You are providing volunteer health services in an underdeveloped country. Only very basic audiologic equipment is available to you: an audiometer and an immittance meter. The budget does not allow you to fly out every patient who is suspected of a possible retro-cochlear lesion to obtain an ABR or any kind of radiologic workup. Additionally, there are so many patients to see during your 1-month stay that you need to be very time efficient. How do you select those patients who need to be flown out for further testing?

2. You are studying a new disorder that is characterized by unilateral hearing loss. One aspect of the disorder you wish to study is recruitment. Which classical test measure would you choose?

3. A patient has hearing within normal limits but complains that loud voices are distorted. Which test would you order?

Answers to Self-Assessment Questions

1. Tone decay and acoustic reflex threshold and decay testing are very quick, requiring only a few minutes per ear and can be performed with minimal equipment. Using a combination of the two methods, you will probably detect at least 80% of the patients with VIIIth nerve lesions and the tumors you miss will probably be the smaller ones. Although this would not be optimal health care, it may be the best approach given the circumstances.

2. The ABLB is a classic and well-accepted measure to examine loudness growth functions and recruitment. If you selected the SISI, please reread that section because it is not a valid measure of recruitment.

3. A PI function would be useful in evaluating this patient. This test would help determine if the patient merely finds loud sound annoying or if true rollover occurs. If true rollover occurs, the patient will need to be further tested for possible retrocochlear disorder, including consideration of possible VIIIth nerve, brainstem, or cortical disorder.

References and Further Reading

1. Brunt M. Bekesy audiometry and loudness balance testing. In: Katz J, ed. *Handbook of Clinical Audiology*. Baltimore: Williams and Wilkins; 1985; 273-291

2. Green D. Tone decay. In: Katz J, ed. *Handbook of Clinical Audiology*. Baltimore: Williams and Wilkins; 1985:304-320.

3. Martin F. The SISI test. In: Katz J, ed. *Handbook of Clinical Audiology*. Baltimore: Williams and Wilkins; 1985:292-303.

4. Musiek F, Audiologic test selection in the detection of eighth nerve disorders *Am J Otol.* 1983;4(4):251-287.

5. Musiek F, Bornstein S. Contemporary aspects of diagnostic audiology. *Am J Otolaryngol.* 1992;3(1):23-33.

6. Musiek F, Gollegy K, Kibbe K, Verkest M. Current concepts on the use of ABR and auditory psychophysical tests in the evaluation of brainstem lesions. *Am J Otol.* 1988;9(suppl):25-35.

9

Noise Exposure, Hearing Protectors, and Industrial Hearing Programs

OVERVIEW: This chapter describes noise-induced hearing loss, including music-induced hearing loss, considerations for hearing protection, permissible noise exposure levels, and industrial hearing programs.

NOISE-INDUCED (INCLUDING MUSIC-INDUCED) HEARING LOSS

Noise-induced hearing loss can occur secondary to even a single very loud noise exposure. More commonly, it occurs secondary to relatively high-level noise exposure over a long period of time. The risk of noise-induced hearing loss is related to both the sound's intensity and duration. Most noise-induced hearing loss starts at approximately the 4000 Hz region on the audiogram, although if the noise is of a very narrow frequency range, as a siren, whistle, or certain musical instruments, the hearing loss may be centered approximately 1/2 octave above that frequency range. Occasionally, an extremely high intensity sound can cause tympanic membrane and/or middle ear damage, or even vestibular dysfunction, but these cases are rare. Most noise-induced hearing loss is sensorineural, reflecting cochlear damage.

Individual susceptibility to noise-induced hearing loss is high and the factors rendering some individuals more susceptible are not fully understood, although genetic predisposition, tobacco abuse, ototoxins, oxidative state, and dyslipidemia may all play a role.

Usually the first indication of noise-induced damage is **temporary threshold shift (TTS)**. This occurs when the patient experiences a change in hearing after noise exposure, but the hearing gradually returns, usually over approximately 16 hours. However, with repeated exposure the hearing only partially returns and the patient develops **permanent threshold shift (PTS)**.

Noise-induced hearing loss may occur suddenly in response to a loud blast but more commonly occurs slowly over time. The first indication of permanent noise-induced damage is generally a **"noise notch,"** which is a sensorineural dip in the audiogram at around 4000 Hz. Although the overall hearing thresholds may be within the normal range, this notch is considered an early warning sign. As this sensorineural hearing loss progresses, the notch frequently deepens and the loss progresses into the lower frequencies. The absence of PTS or a noise notch does not necessarily mean that no noise-induced damage has occurred. Substantial cochlear hair cell loss can occur before hearing thresholds are affected; but currently shifts in hearing threshold are the standard measure used to identify noise-induced damage. However, otoacoustic emissions are becoming more commonly used to provide even earlier identification of noise-induced damage.

If the noise exposure is asymmetric, as in firearm users and some musicians, the hearing loss may also be asymmetric. In firearm users, the loss will generally be worse on the side opposite to the patient's dominant hand because that ear receives the greatest impact.

The patients' complaints will be similar to other patients with high-frequency sensorineural hearing loss (ie, difficulty understanding in background noise, trouble understanding high-pitched voices, "hearing but not understanding"). Usually the patient can understand vowels, but not consonants, rendering it difficult to distinguish one word from another. Noise can also trigger a stress response, possibly exacerbating the patient's difficulties. Tinnitus frequently accompanies noise-induced hearing loss and, for some patients, may be its most persistent and aggravating symptom. Some patients may also experience **"diplacusis,"** which is an inability to perceive a sound's pitch correctly. Diplacusis can be particularly problematic for musicians. However, none of these symptoms is pathognomonic for noise-induced hearing loss and may also occur secondary to other etiologies.

PERMISSIBLE NOISE EXPOSURE LEVELS

In industry, **permissible noise exposure levels (PELs)** are specified by the Occupational Health and Safety Administration (OSHA). The Environmental Protection Agency has standards similar to but somewhat more stringent than OSHA, but OSHA guidelines are most widely cited. The OSHA criteria are intended to protect the average worker from PTS (not necessarily TTS) for 40 years of exposure, for 50 weeks per year, for 8 hours per day. However, these guidelines will not protect all workers from PTS and do not account for any nonwork noise exposure.

Because the risk of noise-induced hearing loss is related to both the sound's duration and intensity, the duration of exposure may be increased as the sound intensity decreases. Therefore, the Permissible Exposure Level (PEL) is based on the time weighted average (TWA) of the noise. The current allowable guidelines (as discussed by Pelton, 1993) are as follows. Note that for every 5 dB increase in the noise level, the allowable exposure duration is halved.

OSHA Noise Standard: Permissible Exposure Level (PEL)

Duration per Day (Hours)	Sound Level dBA*
32	80
16	85
8	90
4	95
2	100
1	105
0.5	110
0.25	115

* dBA is a decibel reference largely used in industry that weights high frequencies more than low frequencies.

Because industrial noise exposure may vary during a work day, a noise dosimeter is sometimes used to measure the TWA or noise exposure in a day's time. A **dosimeter** is a small instrument worn by the worker that samples sound in the environment several times per second over an entire work day and then stores the result for analysis.

If an employee's exposure exceeds the PEL, the employer may choose to reduce noise in the environment, rotate the employees to lower noise environments for part of the work day, or issue hearing protectors. Some employers choose to issue hearing protectors even when the standards are met because, given individual susceptibility, some workers will experience noise-induced hearing loss even when exposure is within the OSHA guidelines.

There are no federal standards regulating nonwork noise exposure, so patient counseling may be critical. Patients frequently do not understand that sound does not need to be loud enough to cause pain or even be annoying to cause hearing loss, particularly over time. A useful suggestion for patients is: "If you have to raise your voice to carry on a conversation easily, the noise may be loud enough to damage your hearing and you should be wearing hearing protection."

Recreational noise exposure has been less well studied than occupational noise exposure but many power tools, lawnmowers, motorcycles, children's toys, and music sources exceed levels for safe sound exposure. Recreational exposure is usually less frequent and of shorter duration than occupational exposure but all of the effects may be cumulative.

Many nonindustrial noises are intense enough to damage hearing. As excerpted from Burtka and Yaremchuck (1997), some examples are:

Sound Level dBA (approximate)

 90 Battery-powered siren on toy ambulance, lawnmower

100 Blowdryer, snowmobile, chain saw

110 Automobile horn, snowblower

120 Jackhammer, rock concert

130 Jet engine at 100 feet

140 Shotgun blast

(A more detailed and precise listing of noise levels for common equipment and exposures is provided in Appendix A of Dobie 1993).

Music-induced hearing loss behaves similarly to other noise-induced hearing loss although it may be more closely related to the particular instrument and type of music played. Curiously, there is some research suggesting that, if a person likes rather than dislikes the music, the amount of hearing loss may be lessened but hearing loss can still occur.

Although some hearing loss may occur secondary to aging, some professionals believe that most of the hearing loss associated with aging is related to a lifetime's exposure to noise. Therefore, some professionals prefer the term **"sociocusis"** rather than **"presbycusis"** when referring to hearing loss in the elderly because sociocusis includes the noise-exposure over the years in addition to aging, whereas presbycusis refers specifically to aging. In studies of populations that were not noise-exposed (eg, the Mabaan tribes of the Sudan), hearing loss is not associated with aging but these populations also vary in other lifestyle and genetic attributes.

ASSESSMENT OF NOISE-INDUCED HEARING LOSS

Industrial Screening Programs

In industry, the requirements for audiometric screening and testing of personnel, allowable noise levels in the test environment, equipment, and calibration are also specified by OSHA. These requirements include baseline and annual audiometric pure-tone air-conduction threshold testing at 0.5, 1, 2, 3, 4, and 6 kHz for both ears of each employee exposed to at least 50% of PEL. In addition, each employee must be evaluated on employment termination unless the last testing occurred within the last 6 months.

To avoid the influence of TTS, testing, whenever possible, is scheduled at least 14 hours after the patient's last noise exposure. If this is not possible, the employee is advised to wear hearing protection until the testing takes place.

Each audiogram must be evaluated and follow-up procedures provided for any employee showing a significant threshold shift. These follow-up procedures are determined by the physician or audiologist overseeing the testing program. However, the criteria for outside referral must be established by outside professionals.

Hearing test results in industry are evaluated not only for changes for each individual worker but also for the company as a whole. To determine the efficacy of the company's hearing conservation program overall, the database of hearing screening results is most commonly analyzed according to the Draft ANSI S12.13-1991, Evaluating the Effectiveness of Hearing Conservation Programs. Basically, test results

are analyzed to determine the percentage of workers whose hearing
worsened in the last year (as a measure of the efficacy of hearing conservation), the amount of simple testing variability as measured by the
percentage of workers whose hearing was better or worse (as a measure of test accuracy).

In an audiology clinic, a complete audiologic assessment for suspected noise-induced hearing loss usually comprises the basic audiologic assessment (see Chapter 1). In addition, many audiologists are
now including otoacoustic emissions because they may provide an earlier indication of noise-induced damage than pure-tone thresholds
alone. Counseling regarding the importance of hearing protection is
also routinely provided. Patients with noise-induced hearing loss are
generally good candidates for hearing aids but, naturally, hearing loss
prevention is preferable.

Hearing Protectors

Because noise-induced hearing loss cannot be cured, its prevention is
critical. Therefore, physicians should be aware of the various types of
hearing protectors available and take an active role in recommending
them to patients.

Hearing Protection in Industry

In industry, hearing protectors are formally called **"personal hearing
protective devices" (PHPDs).** OSHA standards dictate the type and
level of hearing protection required for various work environments
depending on the amount of noise exposure. These regulations recommend hearing protection for TWA ≥ 85 dBA and require it for TWA ≥
90 dBA. However, if a worker has experienced a significant threshold
shift even with only 85 dBA TWA, hearing protection is required.
Hearing protection is also required in any area clearly designated as
"hearing protection required" regardless of the exposure duration and
in any area with unmeasured high noise levels.

The level of protection provided by a given hearing protector is
specified by its **noise reduction rating (NRR).** The hearing protector's
NRR must reduce the employee's noise exposure to ≤ 85 dBA TWA.
For some very high noise level environments, the employee may be
required to wear a combination of protectors (ie, earplugs and earmuffs).

Employees must be provided with hearing protection and replacement hearing protection as needed at no cost to themselves. In addition, an appropriately trained person must fit the hearing protectors to
the workers, provide instruction on the proper use of the hearing protectors, and monitor the workers' use of them. Employers are sup-
posed to provide at least a limited choice of hearing protectors but are

not required to provide any specific hearing protector requested by the employee as long as the protectors provided meet specifications and fit properly. However, employee compliance is higher when they are satisfied with their hearing protectors.

Hearing Protection Outside of Industry

Hearing protection is commonly available as either muffs or earplugs. Perhaps the most common mistake made by patients is assuming that cotton balls or earplugs designed to prevent water from entering the ear are effective hearing protectors. Therefore, it may be helpful to not only ask the patient if he or she is using hearing protection but also to determine the type being used.

Patients also avoid hearing protection because they are afraid that they "won't be able to hear anything." In reality, hearing protectors only attenuate sound and some patients find it easier to listen, particularly over a period of time, with the protectors in place.

For most patients, simple over-the-counter earplugs for hearing protection will be adequate for personal use. These are readily available at most drugstores and usually cost less than one dollar per pair. For patients who constantly lose their earplugs or need to frequently remove and reinsert them, hearing protectors with a string between them may help.

Some patients may need assistance in learning to place earplugs properly in the ears because their efficacy is greatly reduced by improper insertion. For foam or rubberlike earplugs, the proper insertion technique is to roll the earplug between the thumb and index finger until it is tightly compressed. Then pull back on the pinna with the opposite hand while inserting the plug into the canal with the ipsilateral hand. Hold the plug in place for a few seconds until it expands fully.

For difficult to fit ear canals, custom-made earplugs can be made from an earmold impression. Some of these earplugs are also designed to protect the ear from water. Custom earplugs can also be made more cosmetically appealing than standard plugs.

Usually, but not always, earmuffs have higher NRRs than earplugs. Also, some patients with small or sensitive ear canals may prefer earmuffs over earplugs. Earmuffs also avoid exacerbating cerumen impaction or otitis. The primary fitting problems with earmuffs are fitting around glasses or high cheekbones. If the seal around the earmuff is comprised, the hearing protection will probably be inadequate. These fitting problems can frequently be ameliorated by gel-filled earmuffs or earmuff/safety glasses combinations. However, some patients find earmuffs hot or cumbersome and consequently wear them less.

Occasionally, patients assume that their hearing aids can serve as hearing protectors if they leave them in place, but turn them off. However, most hearing aids are vented which precludes adequate hearing protection. If a patient wishes to also use hearing aids for hearing protection, he or she should discuss this option with the audiologist prior to hearing aid fitting. In some cases, a nonvented hearing aid may be used. For the sophisticated hearing aid user, a select-a-vent option, in which the vent may be opened or closed, may be considered. For most cases, however, it is advisable to remove hearing aids and use proper hearing protectors.

Although over-the-counter hearing protectors can be effective, they generally provide greater attenuation of high frequencies than low frequencies, thus distorting sound. They also provide a constant amount of attenuation irrespective of the incoming signal level. Therefore, several hearing protectors have been designed for special applications. For the patient who does not want to invest in custom plugs but simply desires less distortion, the ER20/HI-FI earplugs provide a flatter frequency response than standard over-the-counter earplugs.

For firearm users, earplugs have been designed with a small hole in the center. At low-intensity levels, the hole remains open, but the hole seals in response to high-intensity impact noise. This type of design is commonly called a "sonic valve," but its long-term efficacy has not yet been reported and has been questioned. For hunters, there are also hearing protectors with active circuits. Some of these protectors pass low-intensity sound unamplified but actively reduce the intensity of high-level signals. Others amplify low-intensity signals but actively reduce high-intensity signals. The latter option can be useful for hearing-impaired hunters or those who want to hear prey more easily. Because it has been estimated that the prevalence of noise-induced hearing loss in hunters is approximately 80%, early counseling regarding hearing protection is essential.

For professional musicians, studies have reported the prevalence of noise-induced hearing loss to be as high as 90%. For musicians and music-lovers, several different types of earplugs are available, depending on the patients' needs.

For flat attenuation (ie, equal attenuation of all frequencies, thus no distortion), custom-made earplugs are available. They are designated "ER-15" and "ER-25" and provide 15 dB and 25 dB of attenuation, respectively. These earplugs also alleviate the "echo" or "barrel effect" that prevents some singers from using hearing protection.

Custom earplugs can also be ordered that reduce low frequencies more than high frequencies (eg, to offset partially a high-frequency hearing loss for a musician) or reduce high frequencies more than low frequencies (eg, for a cello player seated next to a flautist). The latter option is often called a "vented" or "tuned" earplug. "Select-a-vent" earmolds are also available allowing the musician to experiment with different settings. For amplified instruments, however, earplugs attenuating across all frequencies should be used.

Protection from music-induced hearing loss can be a complex issue including considerations specific to the instrument used, environmental acoustic characteristics, the musicians' playing style, type of music etc. For a more complete discussion of the topic, M. Chasin provides an excellent review in *Musicians and the Prevention of Hearing Loss.*

Many other earplugs have been designed to be cosmetically inconspicuous or for specific equipment or work environments. Some manufacturers will help select or even design custom hearing protectors for individual patients with special needs.

The primary limitation in hearing protection is obtaining patient compliance before noise-induced hearing loss occurs. The physician can play an important role in identifying high-risk patients and assisting them in obtaining appropriate protection.

Other Applications

Hearing protectors can be useful for a number of applications other than preventing noise-induced hearing loss. Earplugs can also be useful for patients who are sleep-deprived, distracted, or stressed secondary to ambient noise, either continuous or intermittent.

Sources for Hearing Protectors

Because patients and physicians are sometimes uncertain where to obtain specialty hearing protectors, the following is a partial list of providers:

Etymotic Research
61 Martin Lane
Elk Grove Village, IL 60007
(888) 389-6684
(ER-15, ER-25, ER 20/HI-FI)

Westone Labs
P.O. Box 15100
Colorado Springs, CO 80935
(800) 525-5071
(ER-15, ER-25, hunter's plugs) (3 types), plugs for race car drivers and pit crews, orange "safety" earplugs, earplugs that allow you to talk on the telephone yet provide protection, earplugs that are virtually invisible when in place.

Microsonic Labs
P.O. Box 184
Cambridge, PA 15003
(800) 523-7672

Starkey Labs
6700 Washington Avenue South
Eden Prairie, MN 55344
(800) 328-8602
(Active electronic circuits for hunters and shooters)

HEARING CONSERVATION PROGRAMS

OSHA requires that industries with noise levels meeting or exceeding PEL implement a hearing conservation program (HCP). HCPs include not only an audiometric testing program and hearing protection, but also employee education and motivation programs, noise exposure measurement and analysis, and extensive record keeping. A thorough discussion of all the rules, regulations, and legal considerations are beyond the scope of this chapter. The physician who wishes to obtain more detailed information is referred to Dr. Dobie's *Medical-Legal Evaluation of Hearing Loss.*

Summary: Noise-induced hearing loss is a common problem in our society, generally causing a high-frequency, permanent hearing loss. Noise exposure and hearing conservation programs are tightly regulated in industry but are frequently not well regulated outside of industry. A wide variety of hearing protectors are available including those specially designed for musicians, music fans, hunters, and for certain occupations and recreational noise exposure. Selection and proper fitting of the appropriate hearing protection is critical in preventing noise-induced hearing loss.

Self-Assessment Questions

1. A self-employed carpenter is experiencing progressive high-frequency sensorineural hearing loss. His audiologic assessment today shows another 15 dB drop at 4000 Hz. He has been thoroughly counseled regarding noise-induced hearing loss and hearing protection. However, he states that he consistently wears his hearing protectors (earmuffs) whenever using equipment, but frequently experiences tinnitus and TTS. He has his hearing protectors with him and the package indicates a high NRR value. What do you recommend?

2. A rock singer states that she experiences tinnitus after concerts but she can't sing with earplugs in because "of the reverb." They also reduce the treble more than the bass so she has trouble matching her voice to the instruments. Her hearing thresholds are completely normal, but otoacoustic emissions are absent at 4 kHz bilaterally. What is your advice?

3. A dosimeter analysis shows that an employee's TWA exposure is 85 dBA. Does she need to wear hearing protectors?

Answers to Self-Assessment Questions

1. First the fit of the earmuffs should be checked. Particularly in thin individuals, it can be difficult to obtain a seal around the cheekbone area. If the patient wears glasses or safety glasses while working, the seal may also be compromised. If fit is the problem, different earmuffs, particularly gel-filled, may improve the seal. If glasses are the problem, a combination array of safety glasses and earmuffs may be helpful. If there is even a pinhole leak in the seal, protection will be compromised. The patient should also be asked if he sometimes removes or displaces the earmuffs as many workers do when they are hot. If an adequate fit and comfort cannot be obtained, the patient may need to switch to earplugs.

   If the fit is adequate, the patient may need to use both earplugs and earmuffs simultaneously. Many power tools produce very high-intensity noise and the exposure is not regulated for the self-employed worker.

   Also self-employed workers frequently work very long hours, increasing their exposure. The patient may need to be educated regarding the allowable exposure times for the equipment he is using.

If the patient wears hearing aids, he should be advised to remove them or at least turn them off before wearing the earmuffs. If the patient believes that the hearing aids are providing hearing protection when they are turned off, he may need to be appropriately counseled, particularly if the hearing aids or earmolds are vented.

The patient also needs to be counseled regarding the cumulative effects of any recreational noise exposure that he may be experiencing.

2. Although hearing thresholds are normal, the tinnitus and absence of otoacoustic emissions at 4 kHz are early indications of noise-induced damage. This patient's symptoms would probably be eliminated by the ER series of earplugs which do not distort sound and should eliminate the "barrel effect." For a rock musician, the ER-25 earplugs would probably be appropriate given the usual high levels of rock concerts.

3. If she has not experienced a significant threshold shift, she is not required to wear hearing protection. However, if she has experienced a significant threshold shift, hearing protection would be required. If the patient has noticed any problem, including tinnitus or TTS, then hearing protection should be recommended, even if it is not legally required.

References and Further Reading

1. American Academy of Otolaryngology—Head and Neck Surgery/Medical Aspects of Noise Subcommittee. *Otologic Referral Criteria for Occupational Hearing Conservation Programs.* Washington, DC: American Academy of Otolaryngology—Head and Neck Surgery Foundation Inc; 1983.
2. American National Standards Institute. Draft ANSI S12.13-1991: Evaluating the effectiveness of hearing conservation programs. Accredited Standards Committee S12, Noise, Acoustical Society of America, 335 East 45th Street New York, NY 10017-3483.
3. Bohne B, Clark W. Growth of hearing loss and cochlear lesion with increasing duration of noise exposure. In: Hamernik RP, Henderson D, Salvi R, eds. *New Perspectives in Noise Induced Hearing Loss.* New York: Raven Press Publishers; 1982:283-302.
4. Burtka M, Varemchuk K. Variations and pitfalls of noise-induced hearing loss. *Hearing Loss.* 1997:8-12
5. Chasin M. *Musicians and the Prevention of Hearing Loss.* San Diego: Singular Publishing Group Inc; 1996.
6. Code of Federal Regulations. (1994). "Occupational Noise Exposures" (Title 29 Pt. 1910.95). Washington, DC: US Government Printing Office

7. Dobie R. *Medical-Legal Evaluation of Hearing Loss.* New York: Van Nostrand Reinhold Publishers; 1993.

8. McDaniel M. Professional issues in hearing conservation. *Sem Hearing.* 1996;253-259.

9. Pelton PE. Hearing conservation. In: Dobie R, ed. *Medical-Legal Evaluation of Hearing Loss.* New York: Van Nostrand Reinhold Publishers; 1993:174-197.

10

Pseudohypacusis: Functional or Nonorganic Hearing Loss

OVERVIEW: This chapter discusses the various techniques that are used to detect feigned or exaggerated hearing loss including patient history and behaviors, discrepancies in basic battery test results, Stenger tests, the "Yes-No" test, a brief listing of some of the less commonly used techniques of which the physician may wish to be aware, and reference to the electrophysiologic tests, immittance tests, and otoacoustic emissions measures that can be very useful but have already been described in more detail in separate chapters in this book.

PATIENT HISTORY AND BEHAVIORS

Many times the clinician will suspect the possibility of **pseudohypacu-sis** (feigned or exaggerated hearing loss) before the evaluation begins. A wide variety of factors may play a role in pseudohypacusis. Certainly, the possibility of financial compensation to the patient rais-es a red flag that feigned or exaggerated hearing loss may be a possi-bility. Therefore, worker's compensation, industrial noise exposure, disability, or medical-legal evaluations must be performed with the possibility of patient noncompliance in mind.

However, many other factors may also prompt a patient to at least exaggerate hearing thresholds. The child who is not performing well in school or a worker having trouble on the job may wish to have poor performance blamed on hearing loss. A person wishing to avoid mili-tary service may try to use hearing loss as a respectable way to avoid it. The patient who wants more attention or better treatment at home may choose to feign a hearing loss. For example, an older sibling may feign a hearing loss when a new baby enters the family. Conversely, the patient may wish to have less interaction with other individuals and may find a hearing loss to be a convenient excuse. Occasionally, patients will have been previously diagnosed with a mild or unilater-al hearing loss, or with normal hearing and tinnitus, and felt that their problems and the impact on their lives were underestimated by their clinicians. Consequently, they now exaggerate the problems so that "Someone will do something about it."

True **psychogenic** or **hysterical hearing loss** is a much rarer con-dition in which the auditory mechanism is functioning properly and the patient is not consciously malingering but for psychological rea-sons cannot either detect or respond to sound. These patients may not respond to tests in the same manner as malingerers and the clinician may need to depend on otoacoustic emissions, immittance audiometry, and electrophysiologic measures for threshold estimation. Naturally, whenever psychogenic hearing loss is considered because of an appar-ently normal peripheral mechanism, as indicated by normal immit-tance audiometry results and normal otoacoustic emissions, the possi-bility of a central auditory pathology must also be considered (eg, Charcot-Marie Tooth disease with Deafness).

The clinician must also consider the possibility that some patients may have more difficulty than others in following test instructions properly or may be physically or emotionally limited in their ability to attend or respond appropriately. First, the audiologist may wish to check the equipment and reinstruct the patient. But whenever pseudo-hypoacusis is suspected, the best approach is to give the patients the benefit of the doubt, review test procedures, explain that the test results are not valid, that you cannot adequately help them without accurate information, and then enlist cooperation in obtaining good test results. However, it is not advisable to tell them precisely how you knew that the hearing test results were inaccurate because they could simply learn to become more skilled malingerers.

Even before the formal testing begins, several patient behaviors may raise suspicion. Some patients have a very unusual presentation of history and symptoms or may be overly emotional or intense in their presentation. Sometimes the patient may greatly dramatize lipreading the speaker, place a hand behind the ear, or pretend that they understand none of what is being said although they were readily carrying on a conversation with a friend or relative in the waiting room. Some patients will converse fairly easily with the audiologist on the way back to the testing area but pretend to be unable to understand him or her at all once they arrive. Sometimes audiologists will stand behind the patient on the way to the booth and ask, in a relatively soft voice, "Did you have a nice trip in today?" (or similar question unrelated to hearing) and receive an appropriate response. Yet the patient will need to have any question about hearing shouted. A person feigning a unilateral hearing loss may not respond at all when someone attempts to speak on his or her "bad side" even when the sound should be clearly audible in the "good ear." Experienced audiologists are well aware of the degree of communicative impairment resulting from different degrees and types of hearing loss and are usually adept at detecting discrepancies in behavior.

BASIC BATTERY TEST RESULTS

The most common finding in pseudohypacusis is inconsistent test results. Several inconsistencies may be apparent. In testing pure-tone thresholds, test-retest reliability is generally within 5 dB. However, the person feigning hearing loss will frequently have test-retest replicability of 10 dB or greater. Most audiologists routinely recheck threshold for at least one frequency after testing other frequencies as a "reliability recheck." If the recheck result is not within 5 dB, the possibility of a functional component to the loss is suspected.

Patient behaviors during testing can be helpful in detecting feigned or exaggerated hearing loss. Most individuals, when attempting to respond at threshold, will provide a few false-positive responses, particularly if brief "wait intervals" are interspersed during testing. The pseudohypacusic will rarely provide any false-positive responses although he or she will frequently use a grimacing to demonstrate how hard he or she is trying.

For a given suprathreshold intensity level, speech seems louder than pure tones. Therefore, a patient attempting to feign a hearing loss will usually provide speech reception thresholds (SRTs) that are significantly better than the pure-tone thresholds. In a cooperative patient, with or without hearing loss, there is generally excellent agreement between the pure tone average (PTA) and SRT. If the difference is 10 dB or greater, pseudohypacusis should be considered.

As discussed in Chapter 1, a person with one normally hearing ear and one totally deaf ear will still exhibit a "shadow curve" when testing the poorer ear. The shadow curve results when the signal presented to the poorer ear travels across the skull and is perceived in the better ear. For an air-conducted signal, the interaural attenuation is approximately 40–60 dB, depending on the signal's frequency and the attenuation characteristics of that particular patient's head. Therefore, the patient with a complete unilateral deafness will still provide responses for air-conducted stimuli delivered to the poorer ear at approximately 40–60 dB above hearing thresholds in the better ear until masking is employed in the nontest ear. However, the patient feigning a unilateral hearing loss will frequently not respond at all to signals presented to the "bad ear," regardless of stimulus intensity.

The difficulty in matching suprathreshold intensity levels when feigning hearing loss can lead to some unusual audiometric configurations, including odd configurations across frequencies for pure-tone thresholds and/or odd relationships between air-conduction and bone-conduction test results.

If bone-conduction thresholds are substantially worse than air-conduction thresholds, functional hearing loss should be considered. Patients are rarely sophisticated enough to feign a conductive hearing loss which would require them to provide normal thresholds for bone conduction with masking and abnormal thresholds for air-conducted stimuli. However, sometimes the relationship of bone- and air-conduction thresholds is atypical for any known disorder and a functional component must be considered.

Another common finding among pseudohypacusics is unusual results for speech reception threshold and word recognition testing. For example, a patient with a sensorineural hearing loss will generally recognize vowels and miss consonants, particularly "unvoiced" consonants like /s/, /sh/, /k/, /t/, or /th/. The patient feigning a hearing loss may say "hatdig" instead of "hotdog" while the patient with genuine hearing loss might say "topdog." Recognizing consonants but not vowels is not typical of true hearing loss. Further, even severely hearing-impaired patients can generally be encouraged to try to guess the word and when they do will generally select a real as opposed to nonsense word. The pseudohypacusic may refuse to repeat any words or may respond with a nonsense word that has no similarity to the original stimulus. Sometimes pseudohypacusics will even respond with a word containing a different number of syllables. Even profoundly impaired individuals can generally detect the number of syllables in a word for sufficiently loud stimuli.

Another finding in word recognition testing that should raise suspicion of feigned hearing loss is 100% word recognition at 5 dB SL. Another quick check is to simply ask patients if they are getting tired at 5 dB below reported threshold (ensuring that they cannot see your face.) If they respond appropriately to the question, clearly the reported threshold is inaccurate.

There are so many findings in patient behaviors in the test battery that can raise the suspicion of functional hearing loss that they cannot all be discussed here. However, any time that results simply "don't add up," the possibility of functional hearing loss should be considered.

FURTHER TESTING FOR
FUNCTIONAL HEARING LOSS

Many times, the patient simply needs to be instructed that reliable test results were not obtained (specifics should not be provided) and that testing must be repeated. Many patients will simply start cooperating at that point, or on sequential audiograms provide better and better results until true threshold is obtained.

For others, specific tests may be needed. Immittance audiometry, as discussed in Chapter 2, can provide quick and objective measurement of middle ear function. Acoustic reflex measures should be in agreement with basic battery test results. For example, if acoustic reflex thresholds are lower than pure-tone thresholds, a functional component to the hearing loss should be suspected.

Otoacoustic emissions, as discussed in Chapter 4, provide reliable, objective information about cochlear function. If a patient presents a sensorineural hearing loss exceeding 30 dB HL, but transient evoked otoacoustic emissions (TEOAEs) are normal, either the patient has a problem involving the central auditory pathway (eg, auditory neuropathy), has true hysterical deafness, or is feigning the hearing loss.

Electrophysiologic measures, as described in Chapter 5, can also be used to estimate auditory threshold and the integrity of the central auditory system. If immittance audiometry results, auditory electrophysiologic test results, and TEOAEs are bilaterally normal, any hearing loss of ≥30 dB HL presented by the patient is most likely functional, or less likely psychogenic, in origin.

SPECIFIC TESTS FOR PSEUDOHYPACUSIS

With the advent of immittance audiometry, otoacoustic emissions and electrophysiologic measures, tests specifically for pseudohypacusis are less commonly used than in the past with, perhaps, the exception of the Stenger test and the Yes/No Test. Although useful, some of these tests have fallen into disuse simply because it can be more time and cost efficient to proceed to the more objective tests. In some cases, however, these tests can still be useful and the physician may wish to be aware of them.

Stenger Tests

Stenger tests are excellent for patients attempting to feign or exaggerate a unilateral hearing loss. These tests are accurate, quick, and inexpensive. However, these tests do not work well for bilaterally elevated thresholds.

Stenger tests are based on the principle that, if you hear the same signal in both ears simultaneously, you will only perceive the sound on the side in which it is louder. For example, if you put a monaural signal into a set of headphones, you will perceive the signal in the center of your head when the signal is equally loud in both ears. However, if you turn the signal up on one side by only a few dB, you will only perceive it on the louder side and it will have seemingly "disappeared" on the other side. If you lift up the earphone with the louder signal or abruptly attenuate the signal to that side, the softer signal on the other side will suddenly "reappear."

In the Stenger test, either a pure-tone or speech stimulus can be used. In the better or normal ear, the signal is presented at 10 dB above threshold and in the poorer ear, it is presented at 10 dB below the patient's offered threshold. If the patient is exaggerating hearing loss, she or he will be aware of the signal only in the "poorer" ear at a level below reported threshold and will thus not respond. If the patient is not exaggerating hearing threshold, she or he will perceive the signal only in the better ear and will respond appropriately. If the Stenger reveals that the patient is exaggerating hearing threshold, the level of the stimulus in the "poorer" ear can be varied to help approximate true threshold but it is usually more time efficient simply to counsel the patient and retest the basic battery or proceed to immittance audiometry, otoacoustic emissions, and possibly electrophysiologic measures.

The Yes/No Test

This test most commonly works with young children but occasionally works with the less sophisticated adult patient. Basically, the patient is simply instructed to say "Yes" when he or she hears the signal and "No" when he or she does not. Another variation is to have the patient raise the right hand if the signal is audible and the left hand if it is not. By varying the presentation rate of the signal, the audiologist can quickly detect true threshold if the patient actually raises the right hand for the high level signals and the left hand for the soft signals that the patient pretends not to hear.

Ascending-Descending Thresholds

Several studies reported procedures for comparing pure-tone thresholds obtained with descending versus ascending intensity stimuli. For the cooperative patient, both techniques will yield very similar thresholds (within 10 dB), but for the pseudohypacusic, differences are frequently much larger.

Other Tests of Historical Interest

Several tests were commonly used in the past but have been largely abandoned after the development of more objective techniques. These tests are described only briefly here because they are so rarely used. If the reader wishes a fuller discussion, Martin (1985) provides an excellent review.

The **Doefler-Stewart Test** is based on measuring the patient's SRT in the presence of simultaneous noise. The cooperative patient's results will be consistent with original thresholds. However, the pseudohypacusic becomes confused by the varying noise and speech stimuli levels and has difficulty matching the originally offered thresholds.

The **Lombard Test** is based on the principle that we raise the level of our voices in the presence of background noise. Because this "voice reflex" is activated only when the noise level is above the patient's hearing threshold, an increase in vocal intensity indicates that the patient could hear the noise at a suprathreshold level, although the noise may be lower than the patient's offered threshold. However, this test did not provide a good estimate of the patient's actual thresholds.

The **Delayed Auditory Feedback Test** consists of having the patient read aloud a passage without and then with his or her own voice fed back through earphones with a slight time delay. If the level of the delayed signal is truly below threshold, no interference with the patient's reading should occur. If the delayed signal is above threshold, it generally, although not always, interferes with the patient's reading. The Lombard effect was also sometimes observed during this test.

The **Swinging Story Test** can be used for unilateral feigned or exaggerated hearing loss. In this test, some of the story's phrases are presented above threshold in the "good ear," some phrases below offered threshold in the "bad ear," and some phrases to both ears simultaneously. Because the signal changes quickly between the various conditions, patients feigning unilateral hearing loss have difficulty keeping track of which phrases they heard (and wanted to ignore) in the "bad ear," whereas the patient with true hearing loss will simply not be aware of the signal in the poorer ear and will repeat the sections of the story presented in the other two conditions.

Bekesy or automatic audiometry also was commonly used for evaluation of functional hearing loss. As discussed in more detail in Chapter 8, if a patient consistently reports hearing thresholds for puretone stimuli at a much softer level than she or he does a periodically interrupted signal, functional hearing loss is indicated.

Electrodermal audiology is no longer used. It consisted of accompanying clearly audible signals with a small electric shock. The patient would soon learn to anticipate the shock every time a signal was heard and the resultant drop in skin resistance was detected by surface electrodes. At one time, this test was standard procedure for veterans seeking compensation for hearing loss, but it is no longer used because of inaccuracies, patient discomfort, and safety factors.

A FINAL NOTE ABOUT PSEUDOHYPACUSIS

Particularly in the middle of a busy clinic, the pseudohypacusic may seem annoying, time-consuming, and a hindrance to helping the patients who really need us. However, there is generally a reason for individuals to feign hearing loss. The reason may simply be financial but pseudohypacusics also have been shown to have a high incidence of emotional and other psychological disorders. The pseudohypacusic may well be in need of psychological rather than audiologic/otologic assistance and a referral should be considered.

It is also important to remember that many pseudohypacusics do have some degree of actual hearing loss, but the feigned component can render it difficult to evaluate. Therefore, these patients can present a fairly complicated picture.

Summary: There are many ways to detect feigned or exaggerated hearing loss. "Red flags" may include possible financial compensation to the patient, an unlikely history or symptoms, discrepancies between patient behavior and test results, or discrepancies among test results in the basic battery. Fortunately, many tests are available for evaluating suspected nonorganic hearing loss including auditory electrophysiologic measures and otoacoustic emissions that do not require a behavioral response from the patient. However, the presence of pseudohypacusis does not mean that the patient is not in need of some form of assistance and careful patient management is essential.

Self-Assessment Questions

1. You are an expert witness in a legal case. The patient is suing her employer claiming that she completely lost her hearing in the left ear following an explosion at work 6 months ago. Hearing in the right ear is normal.

   After the patient's initial complaint, she was seen by the company nurse who looked in her ears and saw nothing abnormal. After she filed a lawsuit, she was referred to an advanced audiology clinic. For the right ear, her pure-tone thresholds are normal with a pure tone average of 10 dB HL, SRT of 5 dB HL, and 100% word recognition at 40 dB HL. On the left side, the patient does not respond at all to any test stimulus. Tympanograms are bilaterally normal. Crossed and uncrossed acoustic reflexes are present at 90 dB HL for both ears at 500, 1000, 2000, and 4000 Hz. Acoustic reflex decay testing is bilaterally normal at 1000 Hz. The Stenger test is positive for the left ear. TEOAEs are normal in the right ear. In the left ear, TEOAEs are normal at 500 Hz and 1000 Hz, but absent for 2000 Hz and above. Auditory brainstem response (ABR) thresholds for click stimuli are present at 20 dB nHL in the right ear and 50 dB nHL in the left ear. Interpeak latencies are normal.

   You then saw the patient. The otoscopic evaluation is bilaterally normal. When you stand on the patient's right side, she can easily carry on a conversation. However, the patient watches you intently and still cannot understand what you say when you stand on her left side. She states that she cannot hear well enough to continue her job as a foreman on the assembly line and requests permanent disability. What is your opinion and your justifications for it? Remember to include all the evidence for a court case.

2. A 4-year-old child is very displeased about being tested. He will not allow an immittance or otoacoustic emission probe tip near his ear. His test-retest reliability is over 30 dB. He responds for relatively loud sounds but if encouraged to respond to soft sounds he says,"But I didn't HEAR it!". However, when his mother whispered behind him, "If you do well, I'll buy you some ice cream." he immediately spun around and said "I want ice cream NOW!" What is the best approach at this point?

3. A patient has been referred to you for medical clearance for hearing aids by the Department of Rehabilitation Services. You are also asked to delineate any special considerations needed in the workplace, including assistive listening devices. She is a medical transcriptionist who was almost fired for poor quality of work but has filed for special consideration under the Americans with Disabilities Act.

She presents a flat bilateral 70 dB HL sensorineural hearing loss. The audiologist notes test-retest reliability within 15 dB. Her SRTs are 50 dB HL bilaterally and her word recognition scores are 15% and 20% in the right and left ears, respectively, at 90 dB HL. The errors on the word recognition tests are primarily for vowels. The patient complains that she "hears but can't understand." The patient believes that her hearing loss was caused by constantly listening to the transcription machine. The patient is very emotional and cries when talking about her problems.

What is your opinion?

4. A 10-year-old child is doing poorly in school. He presents a bilateral sensorineural hearing loss of a moderate degree (PTA of 50 dB), but the configuration is unusual. The pure-tone threshold configuration is fairly flat for 250 Hz through 1000 Hz and then rises at 2000 Hz before dropping again at 4000 Hz. SRTs are 50 dB bilaterally but word recognition is poor.

Tympanograms are bilaterally normal but crossed and uncrossed acoustic reflexes are absent bilaterally.

The child's results are very consistent but TEOAEs are entirely normal across all frequencies bilaterally.

What is your opinion?

Answers to Self-Assessment Questions

1. There are several classic signs of pseudohypacusis in this case. Even if the patient had lost all of the hearing in her left ear, there should be shadow curve on the audiogram because of the good hearing in the right ear. For pure-tone stimuli in the left ear, she should respond at approximately 40–60 dB HL, depending on stimulus frequency, to signals presented through the left earphone until masking is introduced to the right ear. Similarly, the SRT should be elevated but present until the right ear is masked. The acoustic reflex thresholds for the left ear are better than behavioral thresholds, again suggesting pseudohypacusis as does the positive Stenger test.

   The patient's behaviors also indicate pseudohypacusis. A unilateral hearing loss can be quite troublesome under certain listening conditions and can impair localization of sound. However, in a relatively quiet office listening environment, the good ear should be able to easily detect what is being said, regardless of which side the speaker is standing on. Therefore the patient's behaviors are inappropriate.

   However, the transient otoacoustic emissions and ABR threshold results do suggest hearing loss in the left ear. Given the normal tympanograms and normal acoustic reflex thresholds, the loss is probably sensorineural. Given the normal ABR interpeak latencies and absence of acoustic reflex decay, the loss is probably cochlear in origin, although a very small acoustic neuroma could not be entirely ruled out. The presence of TEOAEs at 500 and 1000 Hz suggests relatively normal (≤30 dB HL) hearing thresholds at those frequencies and hearing ≥30 dB for 2000 Hz and above. ABR threshold evaluation using click stimuli will most closely approximate audiometric thresholds of 2000 to 4000 Hz. An ABR threshold of 50 dB nHL would suggest that the average of hearing thresholds in the 2000 to 4000 Hz range are in the 40 to 60 dB HL range. Therefore, this patient most probably has a unilateral sensorineural sloping, high-frequency hearing loss with relatively normal hearing in the low- to mid-frequency range but of a moderate degree in the high frequency range.

   If her work environment is very noisy, she may indeed have difficulty hearing on her left side because her right ear is effectively masked by ambient noise. Additionally, she may have significant difficulty in localizing some sounds, which may or may not be problematic or even dangerous for her current job placement. If she is in a quiet work environment, she could probably function reasonably well with the good hearing in her right ear or could use a hearing aid, either an ipsilateral fitting or a CROS fitting, to help compensate for the unilateral loss. The selection of appropriate amplification will also depend on her word recognition ability and she has not yet cooperated for this test.

This patient needs to be thoroughly counseled about the need to cooperate fully for behavioral testing so that her problems can be better addressed. Although she does exhibit many classic signs of pseudohypacusis, the audiologic test results suggest that she is exaggerating an actual loss. Of course, it will also be of interest to determine if she had any hearing problems or any audiologic assessment prior to the explosion at work as the loss may have pre-dated the incident.

2. This child may cooperate for the Yes/No test. Simply tell the child to say "Yes" when he hears it and "No" when he doesn't. In this type of case, the child will frequently cooperate by responding "Yes" for the relatively loud signals and "No" for the signals he can hear but that are at a softer level. Naturally when there is no signal at all, the child will have no stimulus to prompt either a yes or no response. This test also avoids a power struggle with the child by not arguing over whether he heard it or not.

If he still does not cooperate, even after all the play audiometric techniques have been exhausted, he may need to return on another day when he is more cooperative or be sedated for ABRs and otoacoustic emissions.

3. As in most cases of pseudohypacusis, the patient shows several classic signs of feigned or exaggerated hearing loss: test-retest reliability exceeding 5 dB, an unusual case history (it is highly unlikely that a transcription machine would cause hearing loss), an incentive for feigning hearing loss (keeping her job despite poor performance), unusual errors on word recognition tests (generally vowels are easier to recognize than consonants), and atypical behaviors or elevated emotional state.

Clearly this patient needs further audiologic assessment after being counseled that the current results are not valid. Further tests would include repeating the basic battery after careful reinstruction but should also include immittance audiometry, otoacoustic emissions, and possibly electrophysiologic measures until accurate information is obtained.

Considering the patient's emotional state and possible impending job loss, a referral for psychological assistance may be appropriate.

4. Although this child may have a functional component to the loss, these findings would be more consistent with auditory neuropathy. An ABR evaluation is needed for differential diagnosis.

References and Further Reading

1. Martin FN. The pseudohypacusic. In: Katz J, *Handbook of Clinical Audiology.* Baltimore: Williams and Wilkins Publishers; 1985:742-768.
2. Snyder J. Audiologic evaluation for exaggerated hearing loss. In: Dobie R, ed. *Medical-Legal Evaluation of Hearing Loss.* New York: Van Nostrand Reinhold Publishers; 1993:48-86.
3. Tate M. Non-organic hearing loss. In: *Principles of Hearing Aid Audiology* London: Chapman and Hall Publishers; 1994:246-252.

Audiologic Monitoring for Ototoxicity

> **OVERVIEW:**   This chapter briefly reviews the most common ototoxic agents requiring monitoring, the characteristics of ototoxic hearing loss, patient considerations, the various audiologic methods used to monitor for potential ototoxic hearing loss, the recommended criteria for determining significant ototoxic change, and the usual schedules for ototoxicity monitoring. Separate chapters describe the individual audiologic tests in more detail.

SELECTION OF PHARMACOLOGIC AGENTS REQUIRING MONITORING

So many drugs and drug combinations can induce hearing loss, tinnitus, balance disorders, or a combination of these symptoms that not all of the potential ototoxins can or will be audiologically monitored. Further, although ototoxicity can cause tinnitus and balance disorders, these symptoms are rarely formally monitored and no generally accepted monitoring protocols exist for them. Therefore, this chapter focuses on monitoring for hearing loss.

The incidence and degree of hearing loss varies widely by the type of ototoxin. For some drugs (eg, erythromycin), ototoxicity is a rare, although possible side effect, whereas in other drugs (eg, high dosage cisplatin), the incidence is approximately half of all patients treated. Some drugs (eg, high dosage salicylates) can cause a reversible hearing loss; others (eg, cisplatin and some aminoglycosides) cause hearing loss that is almost invariably permanent. Loop diuretics can cause hearing loss in adults that is almost always reversible, but research is starting to suggest that the loop diuretic-induced hearing loss in neonates may be permanent. Quinine, in antimalarial doses, is ototoxic. However, anecdotal reports suggest that low dosage quinine (eg, for leg cramps) can also cause hearing loss although it appears to be reversible. In many cases, the ototoxicity of a given drug is unexpected and is not discovered until the drug has been used clinically for some time. This late discovery is particularly true if the incidence of ototoxicity for the drug is low.

Further, certain drug combinations (eg, loop diuretics or cisplatin coadministered with aminoglycoside antibiotics) can interact synergistically, producing substantial hearing loss even when the drugs are administered at levels that would not usually cause hearing loss if administered separately. Similarly noise exposure can exacerbate ototoxic hearing loss and noise in combination with ototoxic drugs (eg, aminoglycosides) can cause hearing loss even when the noise and aminoglycoside antibiotic are administered at levels that would not independently cause hearing loss. Radiation itself may cause hearing loss, but it may also exacerbate the ototoxicity of drugs (eg, cisplatin).

Further, we are just beginning to determine the ototoxicity of a number of environmental ototoxins that are frequently found in industry (eg, organic solvents, gases, and heavy metals). The ototoxic effects can also be experienced by individuals living around the plants if emissions are not carefully controlled. Some of these industrial agents also exacerbate noise-induced hearing loss. Some of these substances are occasionally abused, which exacerbates their ototoxicity. However, monitoring for ototoxicity very rarely occurs in or around industrial environments. Most audiologic monitoring for ototoxicity occurs for patients receiving chemotherapy (cisplatin, nitrogen mustard, DFMO) or aminoglycoside therapy (particularly for tobramycin, or amikacin administration exceeding 1 week or any potentially ototoxic aminoglycoside administered at a high dose or in conjunction with a loop diuretic).

PATIENT CONSIDERATIONS

Determining which patients need monitoring is not always straightforward. Unfortunately, intersubject variability in ototoxicity is very high, even for the same drug and dosing protocol in a group of seemingly similar patients. Many factors may enter into the prediction of whether a given patient will develop hearing loss, including the patient's age, general health, concomitant medications, blood chemistry, kidney function, prior ototoxic drug exposure (eg, aminoglycosides), concomitant noise exposure, radiation, possibly the patient's pigmentation (eg, eye color, race), and many other factors that have not yet been fully determined. Although patient state needs to be considered at the time of referral, audiologic ototoxicity monitoring protocols can be modified even for comatose patients.

In the Veteran's Administration system, sometimes patients can be selected for monitoring by a daily review of new patients listed with the pharmacy. However, in most health care systems, third party payment can be obtained only if the physician refers each patient for monitoring.

CHARACTERISTICS OF OTOTOXIC HEARING LOSS

Most ototoxins cause bilateral, symmetrical high-frequency sensorineural hearing loss that progresses into the lower frequencies and becomes increasingly worse at the high frequencies if the ototoxic drug is continued. Typically, the hearing loss starts in the very high-frequency range (above 8000 Hz) and then progresses into the range of conventional audiometry (250 Hz–8000 Hz). Aminoglycosides generally cause a gradual onset of hearing loss, although careful monitoring of peak and trough levels has reduced the incidence of aminoglycoside-induced hearing loss. Cisplatin, the most potent ototoxin commonly used clinically, can cause marked threshold shift after a single application or no shift for several courses followed by a sudden severe onset of hearing loss. Carboplatin is also ototoxic although seemingly less so than cisplatin. Some ototoxic hearing loss can progress for months even after drug administration (eg, cisplatin, aminoglycosides) is discontinued.

When high-frequency hearing loss occurs, word recognition, particularly in background noise, will generally decrease. The patient may complain that, "I can hear, but I can't understand." Because the patient may be quite ill, the reduction in communication ability may not be immediately recognized as hearing loss unless the patient's hearing is routinely monitored.

Occasionally an ototoxin can cause an asymmetric, or a mid-frequency hearing loss but this finding is atypical. Salicylates, unlike most ototoxins, typically cause a flat, usually, but not always, reversible, sensorineural hearing loss that is often accompanied by tinnitus. Salicylate-induced hearing loss is less common now because the ototoxic side effect is so well known and only occurs at high dosages. However, patients will sometimes self-administer aspirin into an ototoxic range. It has been some suggested that some of the hearing loss and/or tinnitus reported secondary to temporomandibular joint (TMJ) syndrome may be attributable to self-administration of aspirin or nonsteroidal anti-inflammatory pain relievers.

If the patient is immunosuppressed, receiving radiation, or being treated for a respiratory disorder (eg, aminoglycosides for pneumonia), a conductive hearing loss may develop. Although the conductive hearing loss is not secondary to drug ototoxicity, simple pure-tone air-conduction audiometry may suggest an ototoxic change. Therefore, whenever a change in hearing is noted, a complete evaluation must be performed to characterize the change properly.

Although most ototoxins are cochleotoxic, some industrial ototoxins (eg, heavy metals) cause more central auditory damage, and although auditory threshold shift can occur, more frequently, changes can be noted in the auditory brainstem response.

SELECTION OF AUDIOLOGIC TESTS FOR MONITORING OTOTOXICITY

The audiologic tests used to monitor for ototoxicity have been evolving over the years, and the audiologist sometimes tailors protocols to suit the needs of an individual patient.

The first steps in audiologic monitoring are counseling the patient and obtaining a baseline evaluation. The physician should discuss the relative risks and benefits of the treatment with the patient prior to audiologic referral. The audiologist should discuss the possible symptoms of ototoxicity that could occur and the need to avoid noise exposure during and after treatment.

The audiologist should also obtain a brief history of any audiologic or otologic problems the patient may have experienced in the past. If the patient already has a fluctuant or progressive hearing disorder, the results of audiologic monitoring will need to be interpreted in light of that history.

Clearly, the baseline evaluation needs to be performed prior to administration of the ototoxic drug. Otherwise, the medication (and possibly the physician) may be blamed for a pre-existent hearing loss. Because over 10% of the U.S. population is hearing impaired and because many of these patients have not had formal hearing tests, results of monitoring are very difficult to interpret without a baseline evaluation. In general, the audiologist will use the same tests for the baseline evaluation as for the actual monitoring, although he or she may need to modify the procedures if the patient's state changes during the monitoring period. For example, some chemotherapy or infectious disease patients may be better able to attend to listening tasks during some evaluations than others and the audiologist may modify test procedures accordingly.

Word recognition and immittance testing are usually obtained at baseline, but may not necessarily be retested at every evaluation unless a change in thresholds is noted. Because many of these patients are not feeling well at the time of testing, testing time may be a factor in test selection.

Naturally, the basic battery as described in Chapter 1 is essential in monitoring for ototoxicity. Most formal determinations of significant ototoxic change are based on the pure-tone thresholds in the most commonly tested frequency range from 250 Hz through 8000 Hz, which is referred to as the "conventional range." Recall that normal test-retest variability for pure-tone threshold testing in the conventional ranges should not exceed ± 5 dB. At one point, it was recommended that, if threshold changes in the conventional frequency range exceeded 15 dB for one or more frequencies or 20 dB for one frequency, the change was significant, thus suggesting ototoxicity. However, over time, even in untreated individuals, these criteria can occasionally be exceeded.

More recent suggestions have included averaging multiple high-frequency thresholds from 3000 Hz to 8000 Hz. Based on industrial audiometry data, a threshold shift of 10 dB for either the average of 500, 1000, and 2000 Hz or 3000, 4000, or 6000 Hz could be used to indicate true change, although the higher range would clearly be superior for detecting the typically high-frequency ototoxic changes. Guidelines of the American Speech-Language-Hearing Association for determining significant ototoxic change are:

(a) ≥20 dB decrease at any one test frequency, (b) ≥10 dB at any two adjacent test frequencies, or loss of response at three consecutive test frequencies where responses were previously obtained. The latter criterion refers specifically to the highest frequencies tested, where earlier responses are obtained close to the limits of audiometric output and later responses cannot be obtained at the limits of the audiometer. Finally, changes must be confirmed by repeat testing.

Although testing in the conventional frequency range is essential, **high-frequency audiometry** has also become a standard procedure in monitoring for ototoxicity. High-frequency monitoring involves testing air-conduction thresholds for the frequency range above 8000 Hz, usually in the 10000 to 20000 Hz range. The frequencies above 8000 Hz are not generally essential for communication except in the very rare cases in which very high-frequency hearing is preserved in presence of profound hearing loss in the conventional frequency range. However, ototoxic hearing loss usually starts in the very high frequencies and then progresses into the conventional frequency range. Therefore, if changes in the very high-frequency range are noted by using high-frequency monitoring, the physician has the option of modifying the drug regimen before hearing threshold changes in the conventional frequency range. Thus, normal communicative function can probably be preserved.

If the patient's drug regimen cannot be changed, regardless of hearing loss onset, which may occur in some chemotherapy protocols, the audiologist may choose simply to monitor in the conventional frequency range and provide rehabilitation to the patient for any hearing loss that develops. Even when desired, high-frequency audiometry cannot be used on some patients because they do not have measurable hearing in the 10000 to 20000 Hz range even when they have relatively good hearing in the conventional frequency range. This finding is more common in elderly or noise-exposed patients.

Recommendations for significant change criteria for high-frequency audiometry include: threshold change >10 dB at 8000 to 14000 Hz or >15 dB at 16000 to 18000 Hz. Other recommendations include 20 dB shift at one frequency, 15 dB at two frequencies, or ≥10 dB at four or more frequencies across the conventional and high-frequency ranges. However, abbreviated test protocols may be needed for some patients to save time.

Otoacoustic emissions (OAEs) can be used to monitor cochlear function. Research suggests that transient evoked otoacoustic emissions (TEOAEs) diminish in amplitude or disappear prior to ototoxic hearing threshold changes in the conventional range. Therefore, TEOAEs may serve a similar function as high-frequency audiometry in providing the physician with an opportunity to alter the drug regimen prior to impairment of communicative function. DPOAEs may be able to serve a similar function in monitoring for ototoxicity, but they have not yet been fully investigated for that application.

A primary advantage of OAEs is that they require no response from the patient. In fact, OAEs can be used to monitor the cochlear function of comatose patients. OAEs can also be used to monitor individual cochlear function in pediatric patients who cannot be tested under earphones or will not cooperate for behavioral testing. However, OAEs may not always be useful in monitoring patients with pre-existing hearing loss because OAEs may not be present even at the baseline evaluation (ie, if the pre-existing hearing loss is greater than approximately 30 dB HL). As described in Chapter 4, immittance audiometry should be performed in conjunction with OAEs, particularly if OAEs are abnormal, because middle ear problems can diminish TEOAE amplitude or preclude TEOAE recording even in the presence of normal cochlear function.

The auditory brainstem response (ABR) is sometimes used to monitor for ototoxicity in unresponsive or pediatric patients, but OAEs are more commonly used because they are faster, less expensive, and more frequency specific. Generally, ABRs provide a better indication of overall auditory threshold for a broader intensity range than OAEs and can be used to monitor central ototoxicity (eg, for heavy metals). OAEs measure only cochlear function. Some investigators are also working toward developing very high-frequency stimuli for ABR testing so that it can be used to monitor unresponsive or pediatric patients in essentially the same manner as high-frequency audiometry.

Monitoring for ototoxicity is best performed in a sound-treated environment (eg, a sound booth). Bedside testing can be performed, but accuracy can be adversely affected by ambient and patient noise or equipment limitations in that environment.

If any change is noted in auditory threshold for either conventional or high-frequency audiometry, for OAEs, or the ABR, it is essential to check for a concomitant conductive problem. Many patients receiving ototoxic medications (eg, patients receiving aminoglycosides for pneumonia, those who are immunosuppressed by chemotherapy, or patients receiving radiation) are susceptible to middle ear problems. Comparing air- and bone-conduction thresholds and performing immittance audiometry will help distinguish between a sensorineural hearing loss indicating true otoxicity and a conductive hearing loss.

THE MONITORING SCHEDULE

All patients should have a baseline evaluation. After that, patients receiving aminoglycosides are generally monitored once or twice per week, but the risk of ototoxicity is not equal for all aminoglycosides or dosing protocols. Aminoglycosides are frequently administered prophylactically before surgery to prevent infection, but the risk of hearing loss is so low for 1 or 2 days of administration that hearing tests are not usually performed. It is arguable whether vancomycin, by itself, is ototoxic, so the hearing is not always monitored. Gentamycin rarely causes hearing loss, but is more commonly vestibulotoxic. Therefore, hearing is not always monitored during gentamycin administration unless the dose is high or the duration of administration is long. Kanamycin is so notoriously ototoxic that it is rarely used clinically, and if it is, it is very carefully and frequently monitored.

Most commonly, hearing is monitored for long-term (at least 1 week) tobramycin or amikacin administration or for combination therapies because these protocols are more likely to cause hearing loss.

Most monitoring during chemotherapy is for platinum compounds, particularly cisplatin, carboplatin, or cisplatin/carboplatin combination therapies. Hearing loss is very common for most of these protocols, but because the drugs are only administered once every 3 to 4 weeks, the hearing testing is usually scheduled at the same intervals, just prior to the next round of therapy. Testing just prior to each round of therapy is optimal because any hearing recovery from the previous round has generally occurred, allowing the audiologist to determine how much presumably permanent hearing loss has occurred. Additionally, the patient usually feels best at that point in time and thus can better cooperate for testing.

A WORD OF CAUTION

Often patients receiving the types of drugs and dosages described here are critically ill, and their physicians can become so occupied with saving the patient's life that potential hearing complications can be overlooked until it is too late. Obviously, saving the patient's life is of paramount importance, but when patients survive their medical problems, drug-induced hearing problems can cause communication difficulties for the patient and family for the rest of their lives together. Sometimes this time may not be long, but it may be a period during which communication with loved ones may be most important to all involved. Therefore, it is important for physicians to keep this in mind whenever they administer drugs to patients. Drug use may be unavoidable, but ototoxicity monitoring may be critical in helping to avoid communication problems in survivors and in the final weeks and months of those who do not survive.

Summary: Ototoxicity can result from a wide variety of medications and environmental toxins. Ototoxicity can cause hearing loss, balance disorders, and/or tinnitus although usually only hearing is monitored. Most commonly, the physician will be concerned with possible ototoxicity from chemotherapy (eg, cisplatinum or caboplatin) or aminoglycoside antibiotics, particularly when given in combination with loop diuretics. A thorough baseline evaluation prior to treatment is essential for later comparisons of results obtained during and after completion of treatment. Because ototoxic changes usually start in the high frequency range of hearing, high frequency audiometry is commonly used in addition to the basic battery. Particularly in children, otoacoustic emissions are commonly used to obtain individual ear information on cochlear function.

Self-Assessment Questions

1. A 2-year-old child is scheduled for high-dose cisplatin chemotherapy for a malignant brain tumor. The tumor has caused the child to be fussy and irritable. The insurance company requires that the physician specify each audiologic test to be performed or it will not pay for the testing. Which tests do you authorize?

2. A 44-year-old carpenter is scheduled for 6 weeks of amikacin therapy for osteomyelitis. What would be a common monitoring protocol for this patient?

3. A patient complains that every time her "back goes out" she gets tinnitus and hearing loss. What is your first question?

Answers to Self-Assessment Questions

1. It is always a good idea to call the audiologist and discuss the possibilities for testing a given patient. In this case, behavioral audiometry, either COR or play audiometry, may be successful even if the child is experiencing personality changes secondary to the tumor. If it is successful, behavioral testing should be used to monitor throughout the chemotherapy and probably for a few months after discontinuation of the chemotherapy. OAEs, to measure cochlear

function and obtain individual ear information, should be obtained at baseline and should be used to monitor cochlear function throughout and after the chemotherapeutic protocol regardless of whether good behavioral information is obtained. Immittance audiometry will be needed to ensure that OAEs are not contaminated by middle-ear pathology, which is common in this age group.

If good behavioral data cannot be obtained, an ABR could be used to establish baseline threshold data. Because sedation would probably be needed for the ABR, the ABR may not be repeated at every 3 to 4 week monitoring interval. Instead, the audiologist may choose to depend on the OAEs and then repeat the ABR if a change in OAEs is noted and after the end of chemotherapy. The parents should be counseled not to allow noise exposure for the child (eg, loud toys, etc).

2. The patient should have a baseline hearing evaluation prior to administration of the aminoglycoside. Because this patient has a history of noise exposure, it is likely that he has some high-frequency hearing loss. Therefore, it would be very difficult, if not impossible, to interpret the ototoxicity monitoring results without a baseline evaluation, because any high-frequency hearing loss observed could be attributable to either an ototoxic change or a pre-existent hearing loss.

As for any aminoglycoside antibiotic, the physician will need to ensure that the patient is not taking concomitant loop diuretics. The audiologist will have to counsel this patient carefully to avoid noise exposure, not only during the treatment, but for several months after the treatment is discontinued. The patient should also be counseled that, if he is scheduled for aminoglycoside therapy again in the future, he will need to notify the physician that he has previously had aminoglycoside therapy because it will increase his risk of hearing loss.

Because amikacin is one of the more ototoxic aminoglycosides, audiologic monitoring should be scheduled at least once and possibly twice per week, testing at least pure-tone air conduction thresholds in the conventional and high-frequency ranges. If any hearing thresholds change, full testing should immediately take place to determine if there is any evidence of a conductive component. If middle-ear function is abnormal, that problem will need to be addressed separately. If middle-ear function is normal and a significant change is noted on high-frequency audiometry, it is probable that ototoxic changes have occurred. The physician will then have the option of switching the patient to a less ototoxic antibiotic before the hearing loss progresses into the conventional test frequency range and thus preserve communicative function.

3. Your first question should be which drugs she is using to control the pain. It is quite possible that she is self administering high-dosage aspirin and thus inducing ototoxic hearing loss.

References and Further Reading

1. American Speech-Language-Hearing Association. Guidelines for the audiologic management of individuals receiving cochleotoxic drug therapy. *Asha*. 1994;36(suppl 12):11–19.
2. Campbell KCM, Durrant J. Audiologic monitoring for ototoxicity. *Otolaryngol Clin North Am*. 1993;26:(5);903-914.
3. Rybak LP. Hearing: the effects of chemicals. *Otolaryngol Head Neck Surg*. 1992;106:6.
4. Rybak LP, ed. Ototoxicity. *Otolaryngol Clin North Am*. 1993;26:5.

12

Audiologic Assessment and Management of Tinnitus

OVERVIEW: This chapter reviews the most common methods of audiologic assessment and management of tinnitus including tinnitus characterization studies, hearing aid fitting, and the use of tinnitus maskers.

TINNITUS ASSESSMENT

Tinnitus is the perception of sound in the absence of an external stimulus. **Subjective tinnitus**, which is the most common type, occurs when the patient's tinnitus is not audible to others; **objective tinnitus**, which is rare, occurs when the patient's tinnitus is audible to others. Sometimes a stethoscope is used to check for objective tinnitus. Some use the term *tinnitus* to refer only to subjective tinnitus and prefer the term *bruit* for objective tinnitus which is generally, although not always, associated with vascular or middle ear abnormalities or muscle spasm. Although high-frequency or high-pitched tinnitus is most common, tinnitus may be described in a number of ways including buzzing, whistling, ringing, roaring, hissing, "crickets," or "ocean noise." Tinnitus may be continuous, intermittent, or pulsatile.

Tinnitus, is one of the most frustrating otologic/audiologic problems faced by audiologists, physicians, and the affected patients. Naturally, tinnitus patients require a thorough otologic assessment to attempt to determine the etiology and to determine if the tinnitus is symptomatic of a treatable underlying disorder (eg, VIIIth nerve tumor, middle ear pathology, ototoxic drugs). However, in many cases tinnitus is idiopathic, and even when the etiology is known, the tinnitus may not be eliminated by surgical and/or medical intervention. Because the mechanisms of tinnitus are poorly understood in most cases, it is frequently difficult to explain to patients the cause of the problem and to provide a prognosis. Further, the ability to cope with tinnitus seems to vary widely across patients. The impact of tinnitus on daily life often does not clearly correlate with measures of the tinnitus. For some patients, simply knowing that their tinnitus is not the sign of a serious illness is enough to help them adjust to it. Others with seemingly similar tinnitus characteristics may be unable to adjust and report severe life disruption. Tinnitus may cause stress and sleep disturbances, and conversely, stress and sleep disturbances may reduce the patient's ability to ignore the tinnitus. It is frequently difficult to differentiate between cause and effect.

Nonetheless, tinnitus is a common and sometimes disabling disorder. The National Institute on Deafness and Communicative Disorders (NIDCD) has estimated that over 15% of the American population has frequent or constant tinnitus and approximately 10% of those patients experience resultant serious disruption to their lives. Tinnitus is most common in patients over 50. Tinnitus commonly accompanies hearing loss but may also occur in normally hearing individuals.

The Audiologic Assessment

As with any auditory disorder, a first step is a thorough audiologic assessment. As described in separate chapters, the evaluation should include the basic audiologic assessment, immittance audiometry, otoacoustic emissions (OAEs), and possibly the auditory brainstem response (ABR). The basic audiologic assessment can determine the type, configuration, and degree of hearing loss, which may assist in determining the tinnitus' etiology. Immittance audiometry, including tympanometry and acoustic reflexes, can also assist in determining site of lesion. For example, a unilateral, predominantly low-frequency sensorineural hearing loss accompanied by very poor word recognition, normal tympanograms, acoustic reflex thresholds at low sensation levels, recruitment, and unilateral tinnitus would be suggestive of Ménière's disease, particularly if the hearing loss was fluctuant and accompanied by vertiginous spells. However, a high-frequency bilateral symmetric hearing loss with bilateral tinnitus may be secondary to noise exposure. Ototoxic drugs can cause tinnitus in addition to hearing loss. Salicylates frequently cause a flat bilateral hearing loss accompanied by bilateral tinnitus, but both are generally reversible once the salicylates are discontinued. Cisplatin chemotherapy, however, generally causes bilateral high-frequency hearing loss, often accompanied by tinnitus, but the ototoxic symptoms may not be reversible.

Initially, it was hoped that OAEs would provide an objective measurement of tinnitus. However, the presence or absence of OAEs usually corresponds to the presence and degree of hearing loss, as described in Chapter 4, irrespective of the presence or absence of tinnitus. Case reports of spontaneous OAEs in conjunction with objective tinnitus have appeared, but they are the exception rather than the rule.

An ABR, may be appropriate to check for neuro-otologic abnormality, particularly for unilateral tinnitus which may be the first symptom of a vestibular Schwannoma (acoustic neuroma).

TINNITUS CHARACTERIZATION

Tinnitus characterization studies can be time consuming and some patients will have difficulty with these tasks. However, they are useful in attempting to objectify and describe the tinnitus. Tinnitus characterization methodology is not standardized across clinics, and, therefore, exact procedures may vary from clinic to clinic. Additionally, this is an area of ongoing research and is consequently still evolving.

Tinnitus Description

Usually the patient is first asked to describe the tinnitus. Is the tinnitus bilateral or unilateral, localized centrally in the head or even outside the body? Is it constant, intermittent, or fluctuant? Is the onset recent or of long duration? What does the tinnitus sound like? These questions can open discussion between the patient and the audiologist as well as set the starting point for the tinnitus characterization studies.

Loudness Matching

Loudness matching consists of presenting an external signal to the patient and having the patient match its loudness to that of his or her tinnitus. Frequently, the patient is asked to match the loudness of the tinnitus to a tone, presented to the opposite ear, of a frequency different than that of the tinnitus or to a series of different frequencies to obtain more reliable results. Usually the audiologist will start with a tone below threshold and then increase intensity to avoid inducing residual inhibition (see section below), thus contaminating the data. Frequently, the tinnitus loudness match is 5 dB or less above the patient's threshold for that frequency, even when the patient reports the tinnitus to be very loud. However, sensation level is not a measure of loudness, and particularly in the presence of sensorineural hearing loss, recruitment may be a factor. Some investigators have suggested that tinnitus loudness should be considered as a function of dB HL rather than SL to correspond better to the patient's perception of loudness.

Pitch Matching

Essentially the patient is asked to match the pitch of a signal presented through an earphone to that of his or her tinnitus. This match may be accomplished by letting the patient adjust the frequency of the signal to match the tinnitus, or by the audiologist presenting signals of different frequencies until the patient reports that it matches the tinnitus' pitch. Usually this test is performed using signals essentially equal in loudness to that of the tinnitus.

Patients may have difficulty with this task if they have tinnitus that they perceive as an "ocean sound" or other complex signal, although the experienced audiologist may be able to use a variety of signals to help approximate a match. Sometimes a high-frequency audiometer is helpful to match high-frequency tonal tinnitus.

Determination of Minimum Masking Level (Determination of Tinnitus "Maskability")

In this test, a broad-band noise is introduced below threshold into the ear with tinnitus or the ear in which tinnitus is the greatest. The intensity level is then increased in small increments until the patient reports that the tinnitus is no longer audible. This level is called the Minimum Masking Level (MML). Some audiologists consider that the MML is predictive of successful masker use (ie, the lower the MML, the greater the likelihood that the patient will successfully use a masker). If a high level of masking is required (eg, above 10 dB SL) the patient may find the masking signal too distracting and refuse to tolerate the device.

Residual inhibition, or the **postmasking effect**, is the temporary reduction or elimination of tinnitus experienced by some patients after the masking signal has been discontinued. It is generally measured by introducing a suprathreshold broadband noise (eg, 10 dB SL) into the affected ear for 1 minute. After the masking is discontinued the patient must indicate when the tinnitus again becomes barely audible and when it returns to the initial level, and the audiologist records the time until each of these events.

Initially, it was hoped that maskers could routinely provide residual inhibition and thus only periodic masking would be required, but this result does not occur in the majority of patients. In fact most residual inhibition lasts only a few minutes or less. Some patients may even notice a "rebound effect," an increase in tinnitus after masking is discontinued; and others may experience reappearance of the tinnitus during continuous masking.

In general, tinnitus characterization studies can be useful to document and describe the patient's tinnitus and to monitor changes over time with or without treatment. The results of these measures are not necessarily prognostic nor do they necessarily help select an appropriate treatment. They do help verify that the tinnitus is a real phenomenon and can be used to determine it's "maskability." Although these measures cannot always predict the success of a tinnitus masker, they can help select a starting point for fitting, provide the basis for a better discussion and description of the tinnitus, and serve as a baseline to document any further changes.

Rating Scales

Some clinics use rating scales to record the patient's perception of tinnitus loudness, annoyance, or impact on daily life. For example the patient may be asked to rate the tinnitus loudness on a scale from 1–5 with 1 indicating that the tinnitus is very soft and 5 indicating that it is very loud. These scales may yield quite different results from the tinnitus characterization measures because they are strictly subjective and are dependent on the patient's coping mechanisms.

A wide variety of scales exists. Some address the patient's perception of the tinnitus, and others address the amount of disability (eg, interference with concentration, sleep, or hearing), or the amount of handicap (eg, negative impact on personal relationships or employment), emotional distress, drug dependence, or psychological problems (tinnitus patients are prone to depression and anxiety and some become suicidal), or a combination of the above.

Because tinnitus patients tend to show high levels of anxiety and depression on rating scales, these measures may be helpful in directing patients to appropriate psychological assistance when warranted. Some patients even become suicidal and both the physician and audiologist need to be alert for that possibility. Some studies have suggested that some patients' ability to cope with tinnitus may be largely influenced by their psychological makeup and coping abilities, and not just the tinnitus itself.

PATIENT MANAGEMENT

If the tinnitus cannot be eliminated by treating an underlying disorder, some patients may simply learn to ignore the tinnitus, but others may report a serious disruption in their ability to function. In this case, the patient's physician may refer the patient for counseling, biofeedback training, hypnotherapy, or may try drug treatment, although at this point in time drug therapies have generally not been successful for long-term tinnitus reduction. However, treating the depression or anxiety accompanying the tinnitus may help the patient cope. Audiologic management may also be helpful. Evidence exists, from placebo controlled trials, that a "tender loving care" approach may help the patient cope with tinnitus and the audiologist as well as the physician may contribute to this factor.

One step in audiologic patient management is to counsel patients regarding noise exposure and teach them to use hearing protectors even for recreational noise exposure. Noise can cause or exacerbate tinnitus and thus protection is essential. Surprisingly, some patients find that simply wearing protectors seems to reduce their perceived tinnitus.

Although the physician performing the otologic exam will undoubtedly review the patient's medications for possible ototoxicity, the audiologist can sometimes remind the patient to report all medications or change in medications to his or her physician and to report any change in nicotine, alcohol, or caffeine use. Some researchers have suggested that these factors may exacerbate tinnitus. Additionally, it is wise to mention to patients that some researchers suggest that recreational drug use (eg, marijuana) may also cause or exacerbate tinnitus. Many patients are unaware that over-the-counter medications (eg, aspirin) can induce or exacerbate tinnitus. Some patients assume that their tinnitus is secondary to TMJ when the aspirin they self-administer to control the pain may play a role.

Tinnitus masking, which is the reduction in perceived tinnitus by the presence of an external noise, may be provided in a variety of forms although not all tinnitus can be masked. Some patients may simply turn on background music or set the radio between stations to help mask the tinnitus. White noise generators or tapes, particularly of "ocean surf" or similar environmental sounds, may be helpful. Sometimes these signals actually mask the tinnitus, sometimes they simply help the patient relax. At night, patients may wish to use a pillow speaker, readily available at many radio stores, to deliver the signal. A **pillow speaker** is a small flat speaker, placed under the pillow, which connects to the radio's output jack and delivers the sound to the patient's ear without disturbing other individuals in the house.

Desktop maskers are also available. These maskers may simply deliver a white noise or may be able to be "tuned" to be frequency shaped to the patient's own tinnitus to provide more effective masking.

Wearable maskers usually look like a hearing aid but, rather than amplifying sound, they produce a noise, usually a "hissing" sound, that renders the tinnitus less noticeable and is more relaxing to some patients than their own tinnitus. Maskers may be fit ipsilaterally or contralaterally to the tinnitus. Surprisingly, a contralateral masker, even at a low-intensity level, can sometimes provide effective masking for unilateral tinnitus. Maskers can be fitted binaurally, but the masking signal may make it more difficult for the patient to hear external signals. Traditionally, maskers have been fitted in an attempt to mask the tinnitus completely. The output can be frequency shaped to the patient's tinnitus, but frequency matching the masker's output to the tinnitus does not always improve the masker's efficacy. Another approach, developed by Jastreboff, depends on habituation. In this method, the audiologist fits the masker to provide a broad frequency noise that only partially masks the tinnitus. The goal is to teach the patient to ignore the tinnitus. At first the masker is set to mask the tinnitus almost completely, then over a period of months, the masking is gradually reduced until it is no longer needed. This approach is usually used in conjunction with a counseling program.

If the patient has hearing loss, fitting the patient with a hearing aid is frequently a first step in patient management. Amplifying external sound frequently either completely or partially masks the patient's tinnitus, rendering it more tolerable. The audiologist may wish to consider the tinnitus' characteristics in selecting the hearing aid. Additionally, managing the hearing loss itself may reduce the patient's stress level and depression by reducing social isolation and loneliness. Patients with hearing loss may isolate themselves and properly fitted amplification may help reverse this process. Sometimes the patient will be fitted with a hearing aid that also has a built-in masker, sometimes called a "tinnitus instrument." so that a masking noise and amplification are simultaneously provided. One advantage of masking devices, aside from the masking itself, is to provide patients with a sense of control over the tinnitus, which can reduce the associated stress level.

Tinnitus is a perplexing and often frustrating clinical problem. Although assistance can be provided to patients at this point in time, hopefully, future research will yield even more effective therapies.

Summary: Tinnitus is a common problem that is disabling in some patients. Unfortunately, many patients and physicians believe that nothing can be done to help these patients. However, several approaches may be helpful. The audiologic assessment and tinnitus characterization studies can provide useful information not only about the hearing, tinnitus but can also serve to open discussion between the patient, audiologist, and physician. When the tinnitus cannot be ameliorated medically, the patient may benefit from one of several tinnitus masking options or may find the tinnitus substantially less noticeable with an appropriate hearing aid fitting. Both the physician and audiologist need to be alert to the patient's psychological status because some patients with tinnitus become severely distressed.

Self-Assessment Questions

1. A 40-year-old farmer has a sensorineural dip in hearing sensitivity at 4 kHz bilaterally and tinnitus. An otologic/medical evaluation reveals no significant findings and he takes no medications. He reports that, although the tinnitus is loud at times, he has learned to ignore it and it is usually intermittent. He reports no impact on his lifestyle and made an appointment largely at the encouragement of his family. What is your advice?

2. A patient who recently completed cisplatin chemotherapy for ovarian cancer, reports constant loud tinnitus. She states that she is unable to sleep or concentrate. The otologic assessment is unremarkable. She has no hearing loss in the conventional frequency range (250 Hz through 8000 Hz), although the high-frequency audiometry conducted during her chemotherapy for ototoxicity monitoring showed some hearing loss for 14,000 Hz and above bilaterally.

3. A patient states that he has had long-standing tinnitus and high-frequency sensorineural hearing loss for years following military service. During the day, he wears binaural hearing aids that he is pleased with. The hearing aids, not only improve his ability to hear, but render the tinnitus barely noticeable. However at night, the tinnitus is much more noticeable and he wonders if there is anything to help him. He states that he is not overly upset by the tinnitus but feels that he would fall asleep faster without it. The otologic/medical exam is unremarkable. What is your suggestion?

Answers to Self-Assessment Questions

1. This patient should be carefully counseled about the use of hearing protection, preferably by both the audiologist and the physician. Although OSHA regulates noise exposure in the workplace, many people, particularly when self-employed, do not consistently wear hearing protection or do not use it properly. The sensorineural dip in hearing sensitivity at 4 kHz is frequently called a "noise notch" because it is often an early warning sign of noise-induced hearing loss. All patients, particularly those with hearing loss or tinnitus, should be counseled regarding hearing protection because noise exposure is so common. Many patients do not recognize that nonoccupational noise exposure (eg, power tools, lawn mowers, motorcycles, loud music, etc) may cause or exacerbate tinnitus as

well as hearing loss. A good "rule of thumb" for patients is to tell them that, if they cannot easily carry on a conversation in the presence of the noise, they should be wearing hearing protection. Other good suggestions would include cessation of smoking if the patient smokes, possibly reducing caffeine consumption, and avoiding recreational drug use.

2. Several factors need to be considered. The lack of sleep and inability to concentrate may be related not only to the tinnitus, but may also indicate the need for psychological assistance. Depression and anxiety disorders are common in tinnitus patients and may need special attention. Additionally, some tinnitus patients become suicidal but may not volunteer that information. The patient may not acknowledge the psychological impact of the cancer and recent chemotherapy. Tinnitus rating scales and tinnitus characterization studies may serve as a basis for further discussion allowing for better communication and understanding between the clinician and patient.

   Because the patient's hearing is normal in the conventional audiometric range, hearing aids would not be appropriate, but a trial of a masking device may be quite helpful and provide the patient with some sense of control over the tinnitus. The audiologist could review the various masking options available ranging from desktop to wearable maskers. If the patient chooses to use a masker, the patient must be counseled to keep the masking noise below a level that could possibly cause noise-induced hearing loss to which she may be very vulnerable for the next few months. The patient should also be counseled regarding hearing protection to avoid exacerbating the tinnitus. Clearly, this patient will need to be followed and simply telling her that, "There's nothing we can do," could be devastating to her.

3. Because the patient is troubled by the tinnitus only at night, simply turning his radio to soft music or to white noise between stations may be enough to help him. If it bothers others in the house, a pillow speaker or a timer on the radio may help. Desktop maskers or a tape of "ocean surf" could also be tried. As with all patients, particularly hearing aid users, he should be counseled regarding hearing protection.

References and Further Reading

1. Ciba Foundation. *Tinnitus: Ciba Foundation Symposium*. Bath, England: Pitman; 1981.

2. Clark JG, Yanick P. *Tinnitus and Its Management: A Clinical Text for Audiologists.* Springfield, Ill: Charles C Thomas; 1984.
3. Hazell WP, ed. *Tinnitus.* Edinburgh, Scotland: Churchill Livingstone; 1987.
4. Jastreboff PJ, Gray WC, Gold SL. Neurophysiological approach to tinnitus patients. *Am J Otol.* 1996;17(2):236-240.
5. NIDCD Information Clearinghouse. *Tinnitus information packet.* Bethesda, Md: National Institutes of Health; 1996. (call 1-800-241-1044 to order free packet)
6. Shulman A, Aran J, Tonndorf J, Feldman H, Vernon J, eds. *Tinnitus Diagnosis/Treatment.* San Diego, Calif: Singular Publishing Group; 1997.
7. Slater R, Terry M. *Tinnitus: A Guide for Sufferers and Professionals.* London: Croom Helm; 1987.
8. Vernon J, ed. Special Issue: *Tinnitus 1989—A Review of Current Knowledge and Treatment Therapy.* Hearing J. 1989;42:1.

CPT Code Index
for Audiologic Function Tests

(Not All Procedures Have Codes)

CODE	PROCEDURES/TESTS
92551	Screening text, pure tone, air only, 42, 131–132
92552	Pure tone audiometry (threshold); air only, 2–6, 8–11, 143–145, 156–162
92553	air and bone, 6–7, 8-11, 143–145, 156–162
92555	Speech audiometry threshold, 6–7, 8–11, 43, 44, 144–145
92556	with speech recognition, 6–11, 44, 122–123, 144–145
92557	Comprehensive audiometry threshold evaluation and speech recognition (92553 and 92556 combined), 2–11

(For hearing aid evaluation and selection see 92590–92595)

92560	Bekesy audiometry; screening, 116–118, 148
92561	diagnostic, 116–118, 148
92562	Loudness balance tests, alternate binaural or monaural, 118–120
92563	Tone decay test, 121
92564	Short increment sensitivity index (SISI), 114–115
92565	Stenger test, pure tone, 146

(92566 has been deleted. To report, use 92567)

Subject Index